THE FOUNDATIONS OF BALANCE ACUPUNCTURE

A Clinical Reference Manual

Dr. Sonia F. Tan, DAOM, R.Ac., R.TCM.P.

The Foundations of Balance Acupuncture
A Clinical Reference Manual

Copyright © 2020 by Dr. Sonia F. Tan, DAOM, R.Ac., R.TCM.P.

Illustrations copyright © 2020 by Sonia F. Tan
Text copyright © 2020 by Sonia F. Tan

ISBNs
978-1-7361614-0-1 (paperback)
978-1-7361614-1-8 (hardcover)
978-1-7361614-2-5 (eBook)

Published by: Sonia F Tan Inc

ATTESTATIONS

"The late Dr Richard Tan use to often say that he wanted his students to take his teachings past the mental level and into their heart. Sonia Tan has clearly done so and fully embodies the knowledge of The Balance Method. She is a gifted teacher that can lead her students from the beginning to advanced stages of learning in this wonderful art."

—John Maxwell, MTOM, L.Ac.
Senior student, Certified Gold Level Practitioner and
one of the "First Sixteen" of Dr. Richard Teh-Fu Tan, OMD, L.Ac.

"Truly a book for the masses of traditionally trained acupuncturists, Sonia Tan's *The Foundations of Balance Acupuncture: A Clinical Reference Manual* clearly and succinctly lays out the whys and hows of Balance Method Acupuncture. She continues the late Shifu Richard Tan's commitment to his students to not only "keep it simple", but also avoid the common problems of cloistered knowledge and the misleading transmission of incomplete information. I expect similar masterful writing in her future volumes on Balance Method Acupuncture and Chinese Metaphysics."

—Howard Chen, MD, FAAMA, ABOIM
Senior student, the only physician apprentice and
one of the "First Sixteen" of Dr. Richard Teh-Fu Tan, OMD, L.Ac.

"This book is an outstanding reference source for Traditional Chinese Medicine practitioners seeking to build their understanding of the Balance Acupuncture method. Sophisticated enough for experienced TCM practitioners, and clear enough for those with less background, Dr. Sonia Tan creates an easy-to-follow path for those who seek to improve their skills and practice to the benefit of patients. Dr. Tan uses excellent examples and visual aids to make comprehension almost effortless. This book is an opportunity to learn and grow, written by one of the field's thought leaders."

—Nadiya Melnyk, DAOM, L.Ac., MACP
Founder, Wisdom of Health, Inc., Chicago, IL
Author of *Women's Health: Western and Eastern Perspective*

"I have been an acupuncturist for seventeen years. . . . Two years ago, I came across Balance System Acupuncture. It was love at first sight! This style of Acupuncture resonates with me so much that I dove into studying and practicing right away. I was fortunate enough to be among the very first cohort of students at Langara College taught by Dr. Sonia Tan. I now exclusively practice Balance System Acupuncture. With this new Balance Acupuncture clinical reference manual, I am equipped with all the knowledge that I could have to treat patients who come through my clinic within the Balance System Acupuncture realm."

—Fion Chou, R.Ac., R.TCM.P.
Certified Balance System Acupuncture Practitioner

"Sonia Tan did such a thorough and fantastic job with this book. It's not easy to write concepts and explain them on paper, but she did it! I personally loved that she speaks directly to the reader. Being a visual learner, I found all the diagrams very helpful in grasping the material. The patient cases are also very useful to put the whole concept into clinical practice. Well done!"

—Clara Cohen, DTCM Dip., R.Ac.
Chair, Department of Traditional Asian Medicine,
Boucher Institute of Naturopathic Medicine
Owner, Healing Cedar Wellness, Port Moody, BC

"Reading this book made me feel like I was back in the classroom with Sonia! I could hear her voice reminding me that the fundamentals of BSA [Balance System Acupuncture] go a long way in achieving clinical success. As a student of BSA, I appreciated the concise recap of our Acupuncture ancestry; as a clinician, I found the reinforcement of Sonia's clinical pearls invaluable. This reference manual is sure to become my go-to practical clinical resource throughout my BSA career."

—Suzanne Williams, MBA, R.Ac.
Certified Balance System Acupuncture Practitioner
Executive Director, British Columbia Association of
Traditional Chinese Medicine and Acupuncture Practitioners (ATCMA)

"This reference manual has everything you need and more to get started with Balance Acupuncture, from history and origins to practical theory. Dr. Sonia Tan does a great job in compiling different information from historical texts, renowned practitioners, and modern theories exploring Channel Theory. This book is easy to understand yet filled with informational gems, a must-have for anyone looking to learn about Balance Acupuncture or as a reference for any established practitioner."

—Edmund Chin, R.Ac.
Certified Balance System Acupuncture Practitioner

"Sonia Tan creates a concise and easy-to-use guide with *The Foundations of Balance Acupuncture: A Clinical Reference Manual.* The manual provides a brief history of Balance Acupuncture, and Dr. Tan expands on the knowledge of her own mentors and research. She integrates her wealth of clinical experience to pass on her unique perspective. For first-time learners of Balance Acupuncture, it can seem like an overwhelming amount of information since it is not widely taught in Acupuncture schools. This manual breaks that information down with short explanations and diagrams that are easy to interpret for each of the systems. In addition, the clinical case studies help to solidify the reader's understanding of each system. Dr. Tan also provides memorable shortcuts to more complex parts of the different systems. These elements make this an ideal clinical reference for an acupuncturist familiar with the basic foundations of Balance Acupuncture. The reading of the text is also enhanced with hints of the author's own personality within each chapter. The reader can feel the author's enthusiasm for Acupuncture and teaching in the writing. I would highly recommend this book to acupuncturists with the basic knowledge of these systems to confirm their point selections, enhance their practice, or as a refresher on Balance Acupuncture."

—Zaria Valentine, DAOM, L.Ac.

"Dr. Sonia Tan has created a valuable reference guide for the current Balance Method student and a compelling document to spark curiosity in the Balance Method student to be. Her clear writing style is encouraging and friendly. The excellent illustrations and case studies guide the practitioner to begin practicing this powerful system immediately. I enjoyed reading this reference book and look forward to continued use in the clinic."

—Heather Howe, DTCM Dip., R.Ac.

"Dr. Sonia Tan's *The Foundations of Balance Acupuncture: A Clinical Reference Manual* brings the classroom to life and is a must have for the busy practitioner. Sonia's skilled methods of teaching, personal anecdotes, and memories of Dr. Richard Tan light up the pages. This is a great addition to your library and a valuable tool for the new students of Balance System Acupuncture."

—Lisa Curtiss, R.Ac.
Certified Balance System Acupuncture Practitioner

FOREWORD

Dr. Sonia Tan embodies a convergence of factors that have become all too rare in the world of Chinese Medicine today: She is the lineage holder of a family Taoist tradition and a highly trained and seasoned acupuncturist with both the desire and the ability to see beyond the petty goals of self-interest, social, political, and financial gain into the larger picture of the potential of what our art can achieve if and when we work together as a team.

Over the years, Sonia has consistently demonstrated that she can apply her conscience, brains, and woman's intuition to solving both clinical problems and troubleshooting many of the issues that our profession currently faces and will continue to face in the future.

This book, although seemingly simple, is the distillation of all of these skills applied to the beloved tradition that has been passed down to us from our honored teachers. It is an accurate description of several layers of logic that form the basis of our medical practice.

If you are a beginning student or an advanced practitioner of any of the Balance Method schools, reading, contemplating and applying the wisdom on these pages will spread a wildfire of healing through your practice, your community, and the world.

If your journey with the Balance Method is just beginning, count yourself as extremely fortunate to have come to this path in this way.

If your journey with the Balance Method has become your life path and dharma, welcome home.

John Mini, MScM, L.Ac.

GRATITUDES

Rick, my rock, my biggest cheerleader and greatest love. I am forever grateful that when the time was right, you entered my life perfectly, and have been daring greatly alongside me ever since. I treasure your love and support, and it continues to elevate me, and us. I love you deeply.

Prince, my comfort, my joy, my loyal loving companion. Thank you for being my emotional cushion when I need it, and emotional lift when I want to launch. I am grateful for our mutual love for the beach and our long beach walks, because they are the best meditation and healing for us both. I love you to the beach and back.

Shīfù 师傅/師傅 (honorific Master), the late Dr. Richard Teh-Fu Tan—I am forever grateful to have had the opportunity to experience in depth and in person, your charisma, wisdom, and inspiring teachings. I am thankful you included me in the senior student circle, and for your grace and blessing.

Granddads—I feel you every day, helping me in spirit. Thank you for being an inspiring example of the medicine when I was growing up, caring secondary father figures, and for being a spiritual guide for me today as I continue to pass on the beauty of this medicine and metaphysical world. I love and appreciate your wisdom and presence and miss you.

To my parents, Amir Sin-Ming Tan and Athena Ching-On Cheng, and to my brother, Henri K. Tan—thank you for your unwavering and loyal support. You help keep my boat afloat and always do. I love you very much.

To Yvonne Farrell, DAOM, L.Ac.—you helped bring articulation and foundation to my Traditional Chinese Medicine thoughts during my doctoral years, and provided immense emotional support when the weather was rainy and cloudy. Your encouragement to evolve the medicine and pass the lineage on have been paramount to my continuation in teaching and writing. Your leadership and support has been a valuable inspiration to me. Thank you.

To my fellow Balance Method friends and senior student colleagues, John Mini, L.Ac, Howard Chen, MD, and John Maxwell, L.Ac. I greatly appreciate your support and help over the years in shining light and providing clarity and resources regarding the sources, framework, and articulation of the Balance Method. Thank you, and thank you for your friendship and blessings as I continue to pass on the knowledge of the beauty of this brilliant medicine.

To my students! Thank you for continuing to push and pursue me for more, for greater, and for better knowledge. You inspire me to dig deep and give more, and to do so at a higher level. I am happy to lead the elevation and evolution of your skills and talents!

To Kirsten McFarlane, my graphic designer and longtime friend. Thank you for helping make my visions and illustrations come to life beautifully over many years! I very much appreciate your amazing talent and friendship.

To Edmund Chin, my gifted book cover illustrator and bright student of Cohort 1, as well as talented photographer. Thank you for your passion for the method, and bringing beauty and inspiration to my Balance System Acupuncture teachings!

To Joan Giurdanella, my editor extraordinaire. You elevated my book to the next level, keeping sight of my personality, style, and outcomes, and instilling much appreciated industry and professional standards. I graciously thank you for your experience, professionalism, and most of all, our dialogue.

Of great importance are all the teachers that came before me, including those whom I was not able to meet, thank you for imparting your knowledge and innovations to the world, I greatly appreciate your teachings.

Lastly, I am grateful for the amazing medical system of Chinese Medicine and Acupuncture. If it were not for this medicine and its ability to cure me of my own allergies and asthma, I would not have travelled down this enriching path of helping heal others the way that Chinese Medicine and Acupuncture has healed me. Xiè xiè 謝謝 (Thank you.)

A NOTE ON THE STYLE AND TRANSLATION OF CHINESE TERMS

The style used in this book follows a blend of the standard rules of translation, writing, and editing, along with my personal style.

I have opted to translate all the Chinese Medicine and Chinese Metaphysics terms. I have included the pinyin (transliteration of the Chinese characters) in italics with the tone (diacritical) marks, as well as the simplified and traditional Chinese characters, separated by a solidus (/) when both versions are available. For example, *Shīfù* 师傅/師傅 (honorific Master). The exception to this is the Acupuncture channel names.

Most teachers, including myself, use Chinese terms when lecturing. When I teach, I say, *"Yuán Qì" (Original/Ancestral Qi* 原气/氣) rather "Original or Ancestral Qi". When a term is first introduced in a section, I include the pinyin set in italics, tone marks, Chinese characters, and translation *Yì Jīng* 易经/易經 (*The Book of Changes* or *I Ching*). Afterward, I only include the pinyin set in roman and tone marks, without italics. For example, Yì Jīng. The exception to this is book titles, where I have kept the pinyin set in italics, tone marks, and the translation. For example, *Huáng Dì Nèi Jīng* (*The Yellow Emperor's Internal Medicine Classic*).

I use initial capitals for terms that are specific to Chinese Medicine, Chinese Metaphysics, and Balance Acupuncture, which reflects my teaching style.

I firmly believe that including the Chinese terms along with the tone marks is needed for this to be considered a well-written reference manual and textbook. I also want to give readers and students of Acupuncture the ability to see more meaning behind the words in addition to integrating and elevating their understanding of the concepts. I realize that a single word in pinyin or a single Chinese character may often have more than one meaning. The interpretation and choice depends on the context. Tone marks are not only critical to pronunciation but also to meaning because different tones indicate different meanings. Furthermore, some words are just difficult to translate. I am mindful of the fact that there is often no "correct" translation of a Chinese term. Many believe that Chinese is essentially impossible to translate, especially the ancient classic texts. Some say the translations distort them to a view that is not accurately reflective of the Chinese view. Thus, most lecturers generally prefer to use the Chinese word (pinyin) rather than the English translation (myself included), in order to simply hear the word as its embodied meaning, rather than one view point or translation.

Therefore, I hope you, the reader, appreciates the translations and the variations, and are inspired by the deep meaning they represent.

DISCLAIMER

This book is intended to be a reference manual for use in clinics and alongside course instruction. The information in this book is based on the author's education and experience, and is presented for educational purposes to assist the reader and expand their knowledge. The techniques and practices are to be used at the reader's own discretion, ability, and liability. The author is not responsible in any manner whatsoever for any injury that may occur by following instructions in this book.

CONTENTS

INTRODUCTION

Y OU PROBABLY PICKED UP this book out of curiosity. You love the values and philosophy of Acupuncture and Chinese Medicine. This is why you decided to pursue a career in natural health. You've been using what you've been taught in school—with mixed results. Then you heard about the Balance Method and its "instant" results. What?! They didn't teach that in school. Of course not, they taught you the foundations of what you need to learn to start practicing. That's the key word—*start*.

The Balance Method, or as I like to call its evolved form, Balance System Acupuncture, can teach skills that can elevate and launch your practice. This style of Acupuncture is not just effective and efficient, it not only brings the extraordinary powers of trigger and balance healing into reality, it brings them efficiently! Balance System Acupuncture draws information from the ancient classic texts of Chinese Medicine, illustrating how Acupuncture was originally intended to be practiced. This handbook will give new practitioners a window and start into the Balance Method or Balance System Acupuncture, and to give experienced practitioners a reference manual that complements the seminars as a clinical handbook. New practitioners may have more questions after reading this book—you've only scratched the surface—so take the leap and jump in!

The best way to learn this method in-depth is by learning in person, through an energetic, educational exchange of information - come and join me! Purchasing this book marks the beginning of your journey with me and initiates your further evolution as a practitioner. I am excited to accompany you as you take these first steps!
—Dr. Sonia F. Tan, BA, BA(H), DAOM, R.Ac., R.TCM.P.

PART I

Single Systems: Balancing One Channel with One Channel

CHAPTER 1

Origins

THE THING TO REMEMBER about the Balance Method, or Balance System Acupuncture, as I like to call it in its evolved form today, is that it originates from a lesser-used Acupuncture framework of diagnosis that many practitioners of Traditional Chinese Medicine (TCM), or simply Chinese Medicine (CM) as it is originally called, refer to as Channel Theory. Balance System Acupuncture is an extended application of Channel Theory. The late Dr. Chao Chen interpreted CM and Acupuncture classics, and discovered within them systems of balancing channels to treat disorders (Chen, Chen, & Twicken, 2003). Dr. Chen documented these discoveries in a thesis for the 1976 International Acupuncture Congress (Chen, 1976) and in his book *I Ching Acupuncture* (Chen et al., 2003). (Note to book researchers: The original book is currently out of print.) This method of Acupuncture channel/meridian balancing and its use, is also originally documented throughout the *Yì Jīng* 易经/易經 (*The Book of Changes* or *I Ching*) as well as the *Huáng Dì Nèi Jīng* 黄帝内经/黃帝內經 (*The Yellow Emperor's Internal Medicine Classic*). After studying these classics extensively, Dr. Chen was able to determine how to use the *Yì Jīng*, the *Bā Guà* 八卦 (Eight Symbols/Trigrams or Hexagrams), and the *Wǔ Xíng* 五行 (Five Phase/Element) framework, with Acupuncture as described in these classic books, and identify various methods for balancing the channels. Dr. Chen coined this usage "I Ching Acupuncture," which is taught and practiced by other scholars and teachers as the Balance Method (Chen et al., 2003). The Balance Method advances the application of Channel Theory at a deeper level, where a practitioner diagnoses and treats a syndrome according to the channel or meridian affected, rather using the *Bā Gāng Biàn Zhèng* 八纲辩证/八綱辯證 (Eight Principles) and the *Zàng Fǔ* 脏腑/臟腑 (Organs) diagnostic differentiation method, which many TCM practitioners believe is more useful for herbal prescriptions.

The late Richard Teh-Fu Tan, OMD, L.Ac., studied Dr. Chao Chen's works and also the works of Master Tung Ching Chang via Dr. Wei-Chieh Young. Master Tung was a scholar of the *Yì Jīng (The Book of Changes)*, and a traditional Chinese physician from Shandong Province in northern China. He was famous for the miraculous and spontaneous results he would obtain using just a few needles (W. C. Young, 2006). Master Tung's points were a treasured family secret, handed down and refined over many generations (W. C. Young, 2006). Dr. Richard Tan further studied these references from Dr. Chao Chen and Master Tung in the classics such as the *Huáng Dì Nèi Jīng (The Yellow Emperor's Classic of Internal Medicine)* and the *Yì Jīng (The Book of Changes)*, and then refined all of this knowledge into a systematic and logical approach to understanding and applying the Balance Method. He further created his own innovations and systems within the Balance Method, such as the 12 Magical points, which he discusses in his book (R. T-F. Tan, 2003), and I discuss in subsequent teachings (S. F. Tan, 2004–2015). Dr. Richard Teh-Fu Tan calls his whole system the *Richard Tan Balance Method*. It comprises his accumulated knowledge and process of analyzing, diagnosing, and treating.

Throughout this book and in my live and online teachings, I share my clinical experience and unique applications of this style, which I have also verified directly with Shīfù Tan. Since more than one person contributed to the development of this style of Acupuncture, evolving it to how and what we use it today, throughout the rest of this book I will refer to this entire body of knowledge, including my own use and evolution of it, simply as *Balance System Acupuncture*.

Note 1: This book is intended to be a clinical reference handbook. If you have the kind of mind that likes to understand the details of every step explained of Balance System Acupuncture, I recommend taking live course work.

Note 2: You will also see the interchange of the terms *channels* and *meridians*. Both these terms refer to the same concept: the pathway through which the Qì flows in the body. This is commonplace in the CM world, however, the term *channels* is used more often throughout this text because it is a better translation of *Jīng-Luò* 经络/經絡. The most common translation of Jīng-Luò is Pathway or Route channel-Connecting or Network channel. The word *meridian* derives from a French diplomat scholar, George Soulié de Morant (1878–1956), who was the French vice-consul in China, and brought Acupuncture back to Europe in the early 1900s after serving his term, and coined the terms *meridian* and *energy* for Jīng-Luò (Longhurst, 2010). We will use the term *channels* as the choice for a closer translation.

Lì Gān Jiàn Yǐng 立竿见影/立竿見影 (Set Up a Pole and See the Shadow)

As mentioned, Balance System Acupuncture strategy originates from the *Huáng Dì Nèi Jīng* (*The Yellow Emperor's Classic of Internal Medicine*), the *Yì Jīng* (*The Book of Changes*), the Bā Guà, and the Five Phases/Element framework. Drs. Chao Chen, Wei-Chieh Young, and Richard Teh-Fu Tan were able to interpret and apply these systems for use in an empirical way. Dr. Tan also added new innovations to this system (R. T-F. Tan, 2003; S. F. Tan, 2004–2015). Originally termed Balance Method, *Balance System Acupuncture* is a term coined by Dr. Sonia F. Tan, indicating the evolution of the medicine, adding her education and experiences from both implementing and teaching it.

Balance System Acupuncture is a sophisticated system whereby one may achieve "instant" results using Acupuncture through a different lens. Keep in mind, this book does not explain every step and detail of how this system was created and how it works. For that, you need to take a live class.

The idea of "instant" results comes from the classic Chinese text idiom *Lì Gān Jiàn Yǐng* 立杆见影/立杆見影, whose literal translation is "stand pole, view/see shadow; instant effect." It means you should see the results of Acupuncture within *seconds*, not at the next appointment. Fast results are particularly common in cases where you are dealing with pain, tightness, range of motion problems, bloating, or dysmenorrhea. If you apply the system's techniques correctly, you may see a change in the patient's condition right on the table. If you are treating an internal medicine condition, you should see greater shifts at the next appointment. Overall, you may see faster results when using this classical method compared to the traditional methods taught in Acupuncture schools in the last fifty years. If you are interested in comparing the results between the approach traditionally taught in schools and Balance System Acupuncture, you may want to read my doctoral thesis, *Novel Traditional Chinese Medicine Results in Treating Allergic Rhiniti*s, which is available online (https://www.yosan.edu/capstone-projects/) or for purchase on my website. (https://tanbalance.com/books/).

A word about the idiom *Lì Gān Jiàn Yǐng* 立杆见影/立杆見影 (set up a pole, see the shadow; instant effect) and "instant" results. The classics state that Chinese medicine, including Acupuncture, should have this kind of result. This reference is from *Rú shĕn zāo féng zhāng dì èr shí wŭ* 如審遭逢章第二十五 (Chapter 25: Examination of Suffering) in the Han dynasty Daoist alchemical classic *Cān Tóng Qì* 参同契 *(The Seal of Unity of the Three* aka *Akinness of the Three)* (Pregardio, 2011). However, you should be aware of some limitations. Any physical abnormality that cannot be reversed, such as a bone spur that constantly irritates the area, will limit the results. I'm not saying you won't have results. I'm saying the longevity of the results or the ability to get rid of the issue completely will be less likely. This means educating your patients and saying something like this, "We can get you to a maintenance level of 1–2 out of 10 on the pain scale, which means we can reduce the pain and irritation levels significantly and give you improved quality of life."

Historical Origins

Dr. Chao Chen discovered and developed Balance System Acupuncture; Dr. Richard Teh-Fu Tan further refined the system. As mentioned above, the discovery and development of Balance System Acupuncture originates from: a) the *Huáng Dì Nèi Jīng (The Yellow Emperor's Classic of Internal Medicine)*, b) the *Yì Jīng (The Book of Changes)*, and the Bā Guà, and c) the Wŭ Xíng theoretical framework. The *Yì Jīng*, commonly known as the *I Ching* (Wade-Giles translation; or *The Book of Changes),* at a simplistic level, speaks about the cycles of Yīn 阴/陰 and Yáng 阳/陽 and natural life phenomena, represented by the Bā Guà, or Eight Trigrams (or Hexagrams) (S. F. Tan, 2004–2015; Twicken, 2012). The *Huáng Dì Nèi Jīng (The Yellow Emperor's Classic of Internal Medicine),* a primary theoretical text in Chinese Medicine, describes the classification and treatment of Acupuncture meridians with respect to the Bā Guà (S. F. Tan, 2004–2015; Twicken, 2012). Lastly, the Five Phases/Element theoretical framework is a fundamental aspect of Chinese metaphysics, including medical theory, that examines interactions between the five interactions and phases of nature—Wood, Fire, Earth, Metal, and Water—and how they correspond to balances in the body, mind, and spirit—Heaven, Earth, and Mankind (S. F. Tan, 2004–2015, 2010–2011; Twicken, 2012).

Balance System Acupuncture strategy simplifies the complex explanations in the classic texts by concisely and systematically laying out a framework for diagnosing and treating a "sick" meridian. While there is no consensus regarding the time period when the Yīn-Yáng theory and the Wŭ Xíng theory originated, historians do agree that these two ideas were integrated with other major models of Chinese Metaphysics during the Warring states period of the Zhou Dynasty (ca. 1045–221 BCE), marking the start of the common Chinese Medicine practiced today (Twicken, 2012). Using the

Yì Jīng (*The Book of Changes*) with Acupuncture is a system that has been around at least since that time. The famous classical Chinese medicine physician Sūn Sīmiǎo 孫思邈 (ca. CE 581) who is known to have studied the *Yì Jīng* (*The Book of Changes*) extensively (Dharmananda, 2001), says in his book, *Bèi Jí Qiān Jīn Yào Fāng* 备急 千金要方 (*Essential Prescriptions Worth a Thousand in Gold for Every Emergency*), which was written in ca. CE 652, "In order to understand Chinese Medicine and Acupuncture, you have to study . . . and the oracle bones of the *Yì Jīng* 易經. . ." (Dharmananda, 2001; S. F. Tan, 2004–2020).

Fú Xī 伏羲 was the first mythical Chinese emperor said to have discovered the Bā Guà, which consist of continuous lines representing Yáng and broken lines representing Yīn. His arrangement became known as the *Fú Xī Bā Guà* 伏羲八卦 (Early or Pre-Heaven Sequence). During the Zhou Dynasty, approximately 2,500 years ago, during his reign, Acupuncture organ channel systems were introduced into the Bā Guà. Yáng Guà were paired with Yáng channels, and Yīn Guà with Yīn channels. CM practitioners know that each organ system has an original Chinese name, which is, in fact, based on the *Fú Xī Bā Guà*. There is also a *Wén Wáng Bā Guà* 文王八卦, known as the King Wen or Later or Post-Heaven Sequence/Arrangement (some scholars say this is a Daoist arrangement, and did not occur later), that is used for *Fēng Shuǐ* 风水/風水 (geomancy) and lesser known used for Acupuncture channel classification and balancing.

To understand the structure of the *Guà* 卦 (Trigrams or Hexagrams) pertaining to the meridians, one must first look at their origins. In a commentary on the *Yì Jīng* 易经/易經 (*The Book of Changes*), Confucius wrote: "From the limitless *Wú Jí* 无际/ 無際 comes the absolute *Tài Jí* 太极/太極, which generates the two polarities: *Yīn* 阴/陰 and *Yáng* 阳/陽; the two polarities generate the four appearances, *Tài Yáng* 太阴/太陽 [Greater Yang], *Shǎo Yáng* 少阳/少陽 [Diminished Yang], *Tài Yīn* 太 阴/太陰 [Greater Yin], and *Shǎo Yīn* 少阴/少陰 [Diminished Yin], and the four appearances generate the *Bā Guà* 八卦 [Eight Trigrams]" (Alfaro, 2014; S. F. Tan, 2004–2015) (Figure 1).

Essentially, the development of the classifications of the channels and their place in the body came from the ancients' observation of Yīn and Yáng in the natural world, and how they cycle to represent different natural phenomena. The ancients also viewed the representation of these phenomena, the Bā Guà, to correspond to Acupuncture channels, based on their depth or layer in the body that is based on the exposure to the Sun, and the direction the channel travels (toward Heaven, or toward Earth). Further explanation is in the Balance System Acupuncture—Foundations coursework. As with many Chinese theoretical frameworks, this was developed over thousands of years of observation and application.

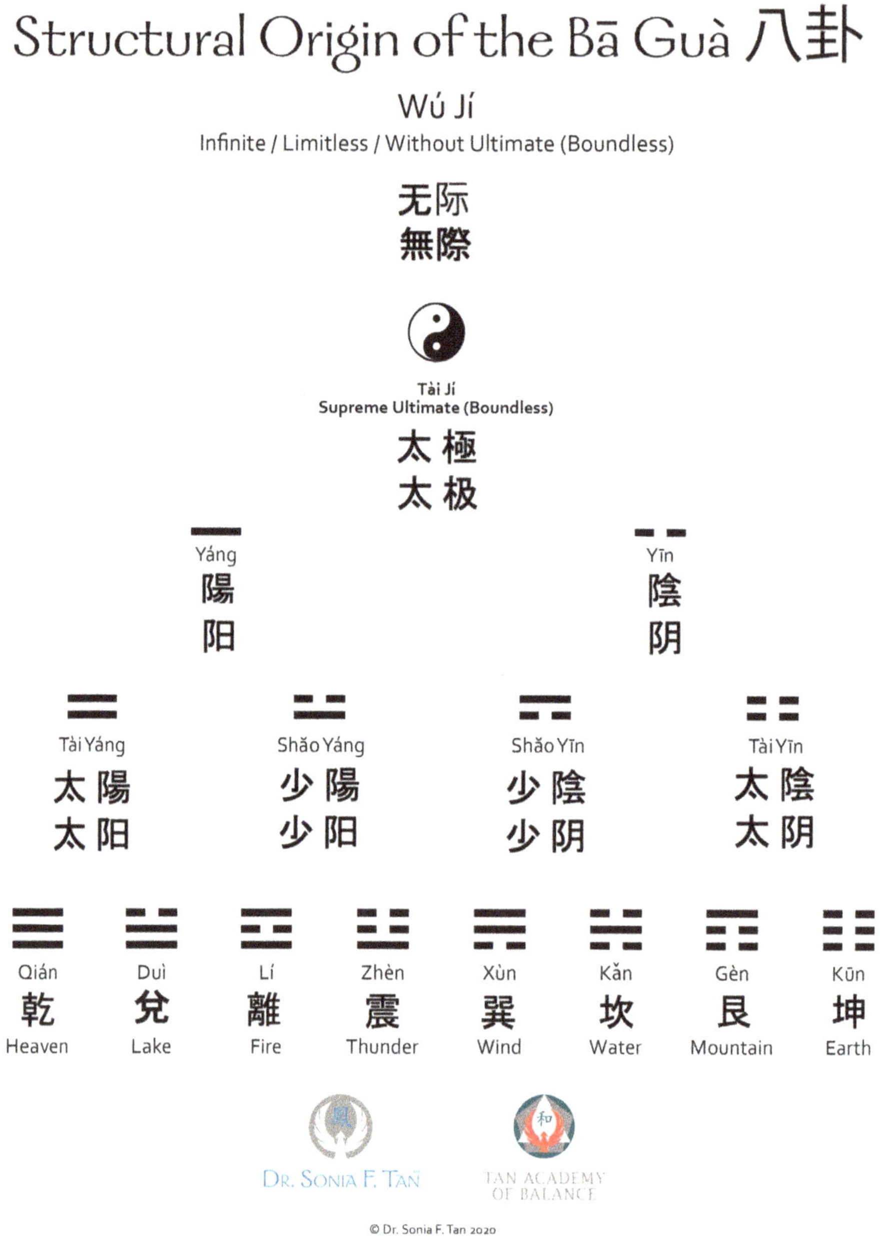

Structural Origin of the Bā Guà 八卦

Wú Jí

Infinite / Limitless / Without Ultimate (Boundless)

无际
無際

Tài Jí
Supreme Ultimate (Boundless)

太極
太极

Yáng	Yīn
陽	陰
阳	阴

Tài Yáng	Shǎo Yáng	Shǎo Yīn	Tài Yīn
太陽	少陽	少陰	太陰
太阳	少阳	少阴	太阴

Qián	Duì	Lí	Zhèn	Xùn	Kǎn	Gèn	Kūn
乾	兌	離	震	巽	坎	艮	坤
Heaven	Lake	Fire	Thunder	Wind	Water	Mountain	Earth

Dr. Sonia F. Tan

TAN ACADEMY OF BALANCE

© Dr. Sonia F. Tan 2020

FIGURE 1

First Steps: Diagnosis and Assessment

Balance System Acupuncture consists of a series of Acupuncture systems rooted in the concept of balancing channels to heal the body (R. T-F. Tan, 2003). This framework uses a diagnostic approach where a practitioner assesses the location of the illness or "sick" area and determines what channels are affected in (or flow through) that area. After assessing which meridians are affected and therefore determined "sick," the practitioner chooses the respective meridians that can restore harmony to these "sick" ones to use for treatment, and their respective Acupuncture points based on this framework.

The first step in Balance System Acupuncture is an anatomical and channel flow assessment. For example, allergic rhinitis is anatomically related to the nose and also the eyes, since conjunctivitis often co-presents with allergic rhinitis. A practitioner should identify Acupuncture channels that flow to the nose, which include the Large Intestine–Hand Yangming channel, the Stomach–Foot Yangming channel, and the less obvious Liver–Foot Jueyin channel (Deadman & Al-Khafaji, 2000). These meridians could be determined to be "sick" meridians, in need of balance.

The next concept extending and used from the Tài Jí is the Six Channel Balance. Within Balance System Acupuncture, there are a variety of ways that a practitioner can choose which channels should help the "sick" meridian(s), and certain strategies for choosing appropriate Acupuncture points. To keep things simple, the basic concept of Balance System Acupuncture involves using a connected channel that can treat and restore harmony to the "sick" channel. For simplicity and relevance, this reference book does not focus on details about point selection and channel diagnosis; that is something that is discussed in detail in live coursework. Rather, keep in mind that this approach is an extension of Channel Theory. According to Channel Theory, when using Acupuncture as a modality of treatment, CM practitioners diagnose and treat according to the channel affected, rather than from an Eight Principles Bā Gāng Biàn Zhèng and the Zàng Fǔ approach to make their diagnoses. Balance System Acupuncture builds on Channel Theory.

To keep things simple, the base concept involves using a connected meridian that can help bring the sick meridian back to a state of balance. Sometimes using the Bā Gāng Biàn Zhèng (Eight Principles) and the Zàng Fǔ approach to make diagnoses, which is taught in modern TCM schools, would aggravate or worsen symptoms. However, as mentioned, in the classical texts of Acupuncture, Acupuncture treatment, if administered and applied correctly, should elicit "instant" and positive results, not aggravated symptoms (R. T-F. Tan, 2007; S. F. Tan, 2004–2015). The efficacy of the treatment as mentioned is called *Lì Gān Jiàn Yǐng* 立竿见影 which is translated as "stand a pole under the sun, and you should immediately see its shadow" (R. T-F. Tan, 2007). This means that one should see instant and positive results with Acupuncture, not slow or worse results, when applied correctly (S. F. Tan, 2004–2015; R. T-F. Tan, 2007). This idea is based on six different systems of balancing a "sick" meridian with other meridians that are energetically connected to it.

Let's explore this further!

CHAPTER 2

System I: Míng 名 (Name)

ABOUT TWO THOUSAND YEARS ago, ancient elders of China figured out how to explain phenomena in Heavens or the Universe and seasonal changes on Earth in a simple way, using *Yáo* 爻 (bar line) representing Yīn (broken bar line) and Yáng (solid bar line). These solid and broken lines, which compose the *Bā Guà* 八卦 (Eight Trigrams or Hexagrams), are also the basis of the Chinese metaphysical practices—Fēng Shuǐ 风水/風水 (geomancy) and Astrology. In fact, at one point in history, ancient Chinese doctors knew how to practice all three areas of Chinese metaphysics (Astrology, Acupuncture, and Fēng Shuǐ, following the philosophy of the *Sān Cái* 三才 (Three Essences) – *Tiān* 天 *Rén* 人 *Dì* 地 – which means to have harmony in life, we must be mindful of the Three Essences: between Heaven (Tiān 天) and Earth (Dì 地), there is humankind (Rén 人). This concept means that we must find a way to be balanced with all these forces of energy, and its applications, interacting on us—Humans—in the middle of it all.

If we look at this concept further, it is attached to each concept for a reason. The Heavens is the energy from the Universe, which is also associated with Chinese Astrology—our "DNA Qì" that we are born with as I like to say (not the same as *Yuán*-Ancestral/Original *Qì* 原气/氣). This Qì we inhale from the Universe at the time we are born makes up who we are and defines our constitution, personality characteristics, and our destiny. The energy from Earth involves the seasonal changes in nature and is associated with Fēng Shuǐ, which involves living in harmony with the environment. I like to call it "environmental design." Lastly, there is Humankind, centered in the middle of this—Heaven and Earth, absorbing and exchanging energy. Just like the moon can pull tides and the ocean, energy can affect humans—after all, roughly 55 to 60 percent of the adult human body is made of fluids and therefore can be affected by energy just like water is pulled to change the tides. A true Chinese metaphysical doctor would know how to practice in all three areas, because they would need to properly advise patients based on their individual "DNA Qì" (Astrology), the uniquely appropriate environmental design they live in (Fēng Shuǐ), and the uniquely appropriate Chinese Medicine and Acupuncture to restore and balance their health (Humankind). These are long historically known to all Chinese metaphysicians as the Three Essences—Sān Cái 三才: Astrology, Fēng Shuǐ, and Humankind.

When we can dive into this further, we can see the representation of the Sān Cái—Three Essences in our body via the Acupuncture channels. Our body reflects this divine balance. Look at how the true Chinese anatomical man is positioned: palms facing medial and hands to the sky. All the Yáng channels start at the Heavens (the sky) and move toward the Earth (the ground). All the Yīn channels start at the Earth (the ground) and move toward the Heavens. Living between these intersections of energy is our body—humans. Thus, our body illustrates this concept that between Heaven and Earth, there is Humankind, and when we are doing Acupuncture, we are intending to create balance and harmony of these Three Essences, within the patient's body. Not just interesting, let's admit it and say exciting!

It began when the ancients observed how the state of the Universe is, limitless, and then observed that we in fact have a polarity that co-exists within the Universe—Yīn and Yáng—Tài Jí (Figure 1). As you learned in school, Yīn and Yáng must exist together in order for there to be balance. This dual relationship has many scenarios with respect to phenomena and balance. Figure 1 illustrates the possible scenarios on a micro and macro scale. Given three possible scenarios (micro and macro scale comparisons) with a base of a dual relationship, there are eight possible outcomes (2^3): the Bā Guà (Figure 1).

The discovery of the Bā Guà happened approximately two thousand years ago, which is when Chinese thinkers first described and assigned the Five Phases/Interactions, or Elements as they are commonly referred to. Also at this time, organ channel systems were assigned to each Guà, based on the energetics contained in each one as shown in Figure 1. You can see that each Guà in the Bā Guà has three *Yáo* 爻 (bar lines). The most and purest amount of Yáng (three solid lines) is assigned to the Du vessel. In the animal kingdom, Yáng channels are the ones that are the most exposed to the Sun. Imagine an animal on all fours, and you will see what channels are more exposed to the Sun—this correlation is also true for the human body. Furthermore, all the Yīn channels are least exposed to the Sun, protecting the interior. Even further, within the Yáng and Yīn channels, they are layered from the most superficial to the deepest. Look at the Yīn channels on the arm as you hold your hand out to the side, palms facing anterior. The Taiyin channel is closer to the Sun, and the Shaoyin channel is least exposed to Sun. They are named that way for a reason! Where their layer lies in the body and its exposure to the exterior determines their name. From here, an important concept to remember is: a) each bar or line is called a Yáo, b) the Yīn bars (broken line) have an affinity or attraction to the Yáng bars (solid line), in order for there to be balance, and vice versa. They are attracted to each other, and want to find each other to establish balance. Hence, they will seek their exact opposite Guà in order to find balance (see Figure 2). You have just observed your first Balance System! This system is called Míng 名, which means "Name."

Dr. Richard Teh-Fu Tan decided to assign numbers to the systems in order to create a logical meaningful way to memorize them. This system, Míng–Name, is also referred to as System I (using the Roman numeral). Dr. Richard Tan assigned odd numbers to systems for a reason: they must be treated *only* on the contralateral side of the body! In addition, any strategy or treatment system is assigned the use of a Roman numeral for visual distinction. In System I: Míng–Name, you treat by using the balancing channel of the same named channel, then switch the limb (go from Hand to Foot), and treat on the contralateral side. For example, if the Hand Taiyang–Small Intestine channel is "sick" or "blocked," then when using System I, the balancing channel that can send a healing response to this blocked channel is the Foot Taiyang–Bladder channel. Treatment effect is only from the contralateral side.

A word about the term *Single Systems*. This is a term I developed, as a way to make more of a clear distinction and understanding of its use, function, and intended outcome. Shīfù Tan referred to this as Acupuncture 1,2,3.

SYSTEM #1

MÍNG 名 → SAME CHANNEL NAME

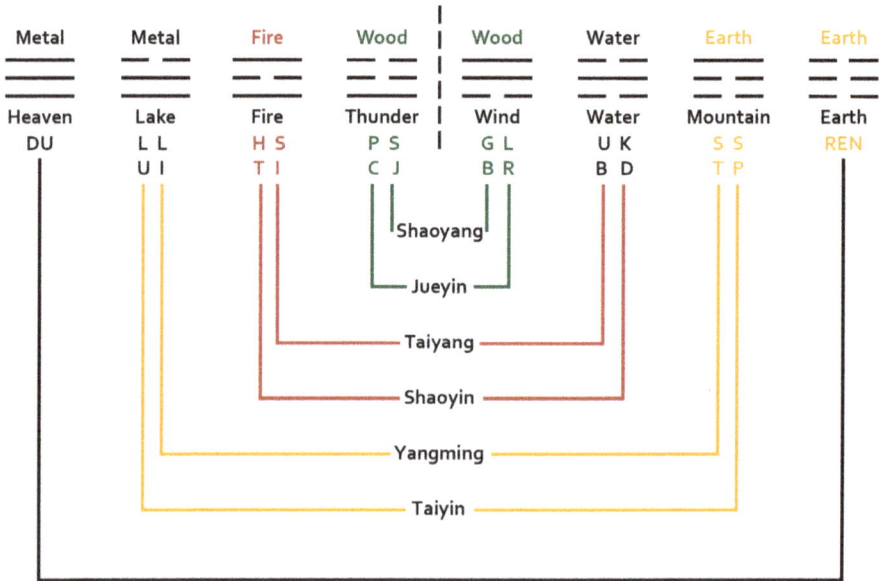

Metal	Metal	Fire	Wood	Wood	Water	Earth	Earth
Heaven	Lake	Fire	Thunder	Wind	Water	Mountain	Earth
DU	L L	H S	P S	G L	U K	S S	REN
	U I	T I	C J	B R	B D	T P	

Shaoyang

Jueyin

Taiyang

Shaoyin

Yangming

Taiyin

Same channel name.

Switch limbs.

Contralateral treatment.

Dr. Sonia F. Tan

TAN ACADEMY OF BALANCE

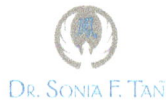

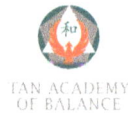

© Dr. Sonia F. Tan 2020

FIGURE 2

CHAPTER 3

Holography:
The Mirror-Image Systems

I KNOW WHAT YOU ARE thinking. *So I found the balancing channel, now where do I go, what points on the channel do I use?* Here's where we get into the holographic (imaging) maps of the main micro systems used in Balance System Acupuncture.

The concept of holography, or imaging and mirroring, comes from the theory of *Tài Jí* 太极/太極 and *Yuán Qì* 原气/氣 (Ancestral/Original Qi) from the *Yì Jīng* 易经/易經 (*The Book of Changes*) (Twicken, 2012). One scholar, Dr. Wei-Chieh Young refers to holography as *Tǐ Yìng Quán Xī* 体应全息/體應全息 (Tissue Correspondence Holographic Model) and explains that this concept is rooted and referenced in the *Huáng Dì Nèi Jīng* 黄帝内经/黃帝內經 (*The Yellow Emperor's Internal Medicine Classic*) (Young, Chang, & Morris, 2003). He further discussed holography in his book *Lectures on Tung's Acupuncture Therapeutic System* (Young, 2008).

Holography is a mapping system that is termed *Quán Xī* 全息 in Chinese, which means "complete message," "whole information," "holographic," or "microsystem." some practitioners consider Quán Xī to be the core theoretical basis for Acupuncture (Young et al., 2003). Remember, we mentioned the Chinese believe that there is a relationship between Tiān 天 (Heaven), also referred to as "the Universe" and Rén 人(Man), also referred to as "a person or human." In fact, Confucian scholars state that "man exists in the Universe, and the Universe exists in man" (Alfaro, 2014). Many areas of CM believe that human body parts are miniature organic structures of the whole body, as observed in auricular acupuncture, reflexology, and tongue diagnosis. The Tài Jí of the human body identifies the umbilicus as the core, or center, of the body. Extending from there, a practitioner can view the arms and legs as representations of the torso, as well as representations of the face, with the umbilicus and eyes equaling the level of elbows and knees (see Figures 3, 4, 5, and 6). What this represents is a system for choosing points on a particular channel based on its corresponding "image." This concept of Holography, or Mirror and Imaging, is one of the foundations of Balance System Acupuncture. The choice of which channel to use to balance and send a healing response, is of primary importance, as well as choosing the appropriate side of the body and the correct mirror-image site.

Figures 3 to 10 are the most common mirror-image systems "maps" used in Balance System Acupuncture. While there are more micro systems out there, I've included the most commonly used ones. You may learn more through courses, online, or colleagues, and that's fine, use them in a Balance System Acupuncture way for improved clinical outcomes.

Here is a general guideline for choosing which mirror-image to use:

1. Select the area that is the most anatomically like the "sick" area.
2. Choose an area that has a larger image area to work with. With a larger target area to work with, you are more likely access the exact epicenter of blockage you are aiming to unblock, to access channel flow, and to generate a healing response.
3. You can choose to overlap images and treat many areas of the body with one mirror-image area.
4. You may want to switch mirror-images or Systems over time, to trigger the body to have a greater healing response and to improve your patient's healing trajectory.

ILLUSTRATIONS OF THE IMAGING CONCEPT
APPLIED IN THE BALANCE SYSTEM

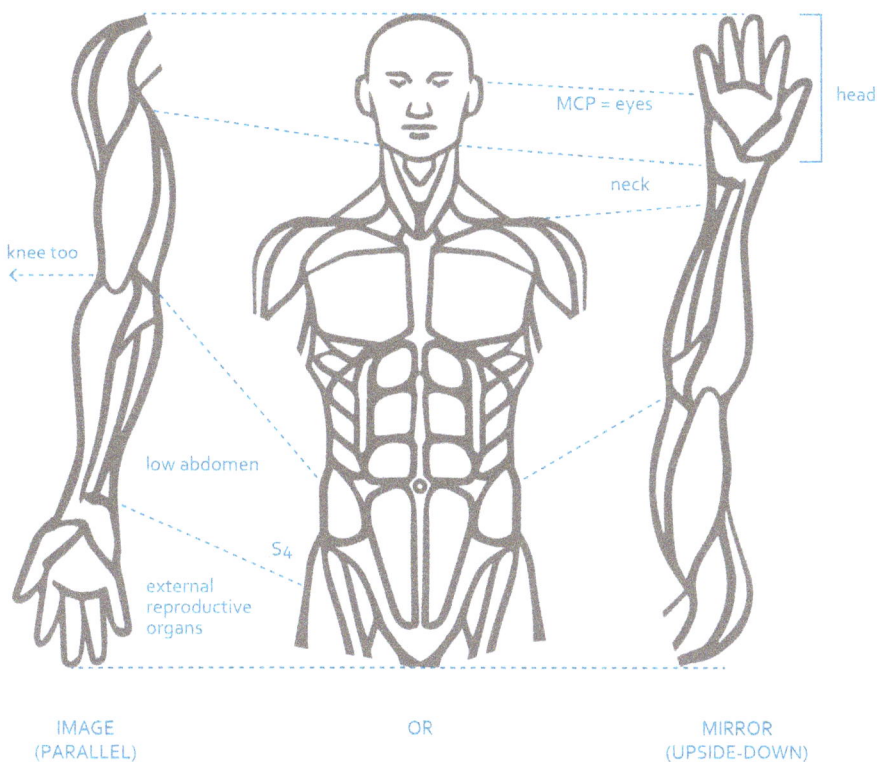

MCP = eyes

head

neck

knee too

low abdomen

S4

external
reproductive
organs

IMAGE
(PARALLEL)

OR

MIRROR
(UPSIDE-DOWN)

These are approximate guidelines and will vary according to the proportions of the human body.

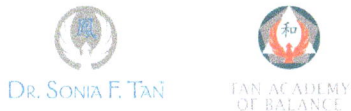

DR. SONIA F. TAN

TAN ACADEMY
OF BALANCE

FIGURE 3

ILLUSTRATIONS OF THE IMAGING CONCEPT
APPLIED IN THE BALANCE SYSTEM

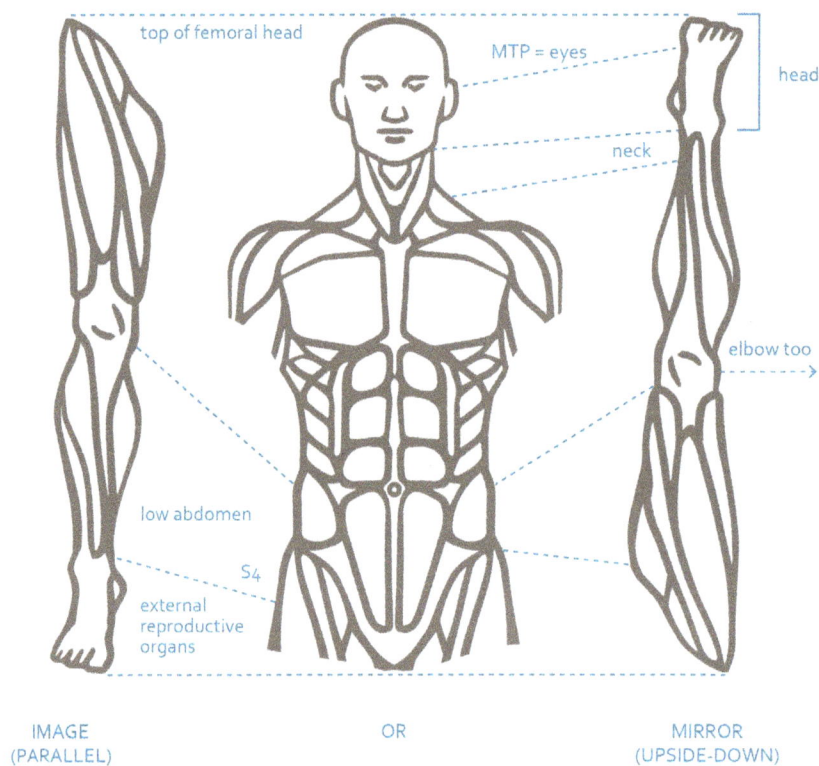

top of femoral head

MTP = eyes

head

neck

elbow too

low abdomen

S4

external
reproductive
organs

IMAGE
(PARALLEL)

OR

MIRROR
(UPSIDE-DOWN)

These are approximate guidelines and will vary according to the proportions of the human body.

DR. SONIA F. TAN

TAN ACADEMY
OF BALANCE

© Dr. Sonia F. Tan 2020

FIGURE 4

ILLUSTRATIONS OF THE IMAGING CONCEPT
APPLIED IN THE BALANCE SYSTEM

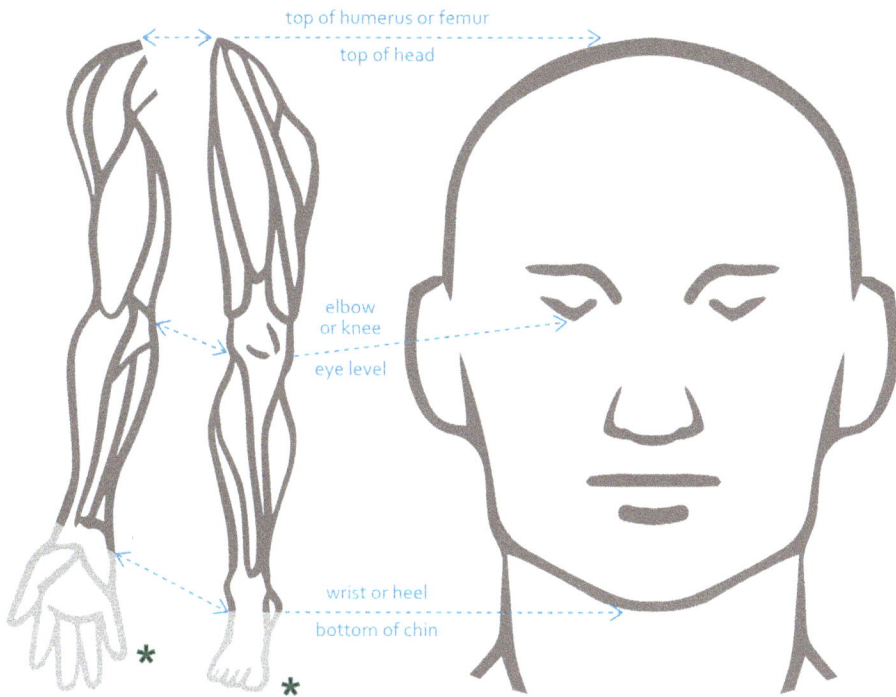

top of humerus or femur

top of head

elbow
or knee

eye level

wrist or heel

bottom of chin

* also can flip the image

These are approximate guidelines and will vary according to the proportions of the human body.

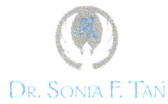

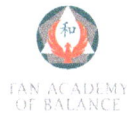

Dr. Sonia F. Tan

TAN ACADEMY OF BALANCE

© Dr. Sonia F. Tan 2020

FIGURE 5

ILLUSTRATIONS OF THE IMAGING CONCEPT
APPLIED IN THE BALANCE SYSTEM

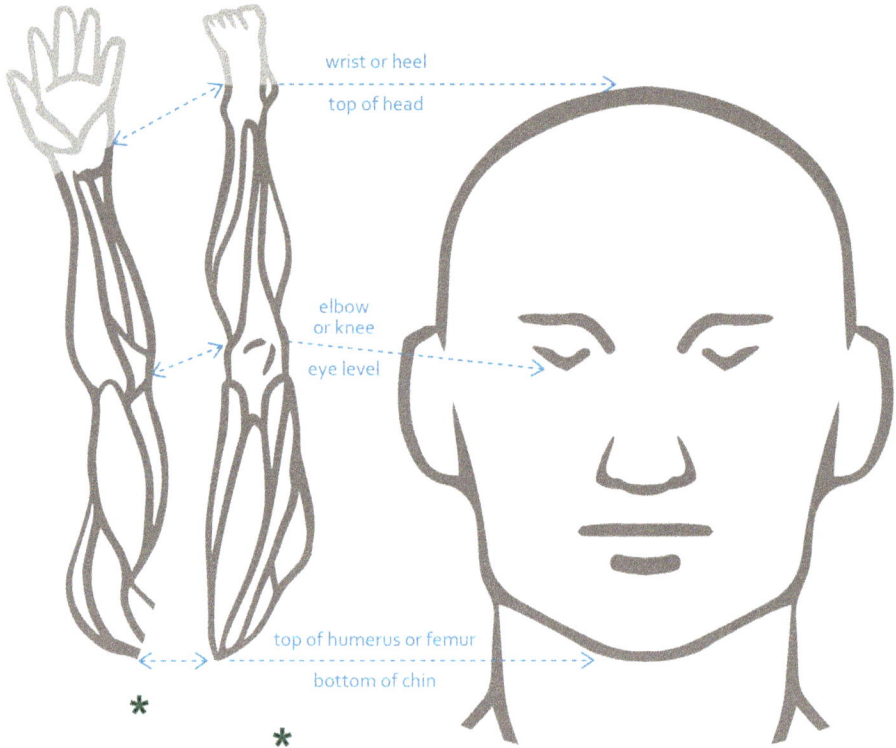

wrist or heel

top of head

elbow
or knee

eye level

top of humerus or femur

bottom of chin

* also can flip the image

These are approximate guidelines and will vary according to the proportions of the human body.

DR. SONIA F. TAN

TAN ACADEMY
OF BALANCE

© Dr. Sonia F. Tan 2020

FIGURE 6

ILLUSTRATIONS OF THE IMAGING CONCEPT
APPLIED IN THE BALANCE SYSTEM

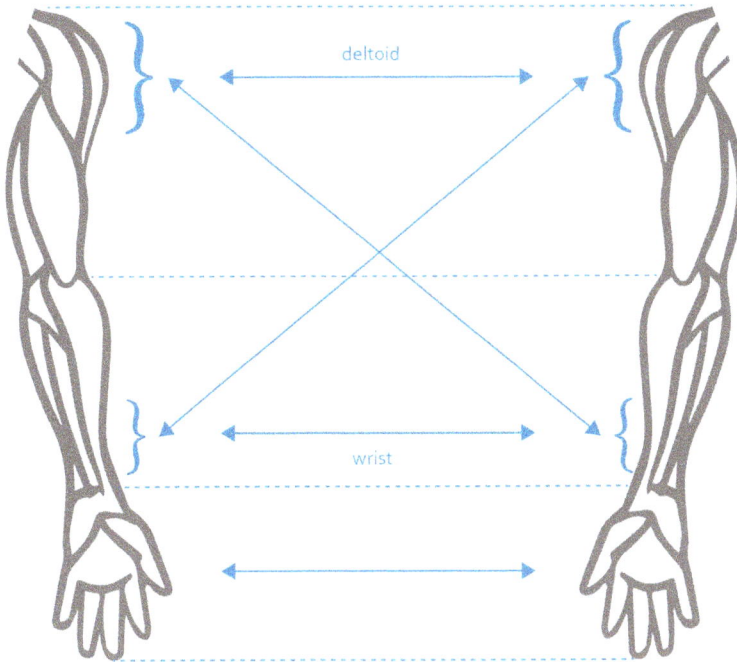

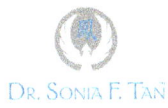

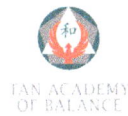

deltoid

wrist

DR. SONIA F. TAN

TAN ACADEMY
OF BALANCE

© Dr. Sonia F. Tan 2020

FIGURE 7

ILLUSTRATIONS OF THE IMAGING CONCEPT
APPLIED IN THE BALANCE SYSTEM

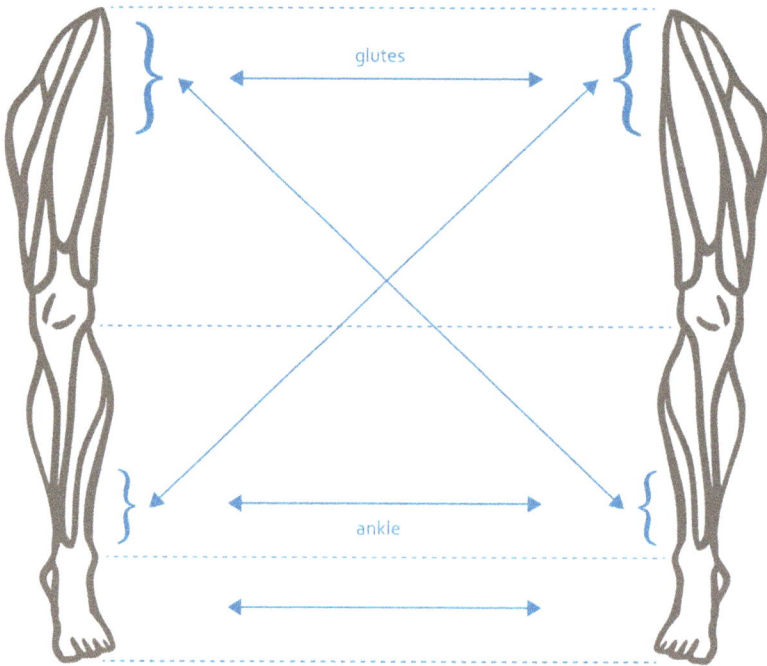

glutes

ankle

DR. SONIA F. TAN

TAN ACADEMY
OF BALANCE

FIGURE 8

ILLUSTRATIONS OF THE IMAGING CONCEPT
APPLIED IN THE BALANCE SYSTEM

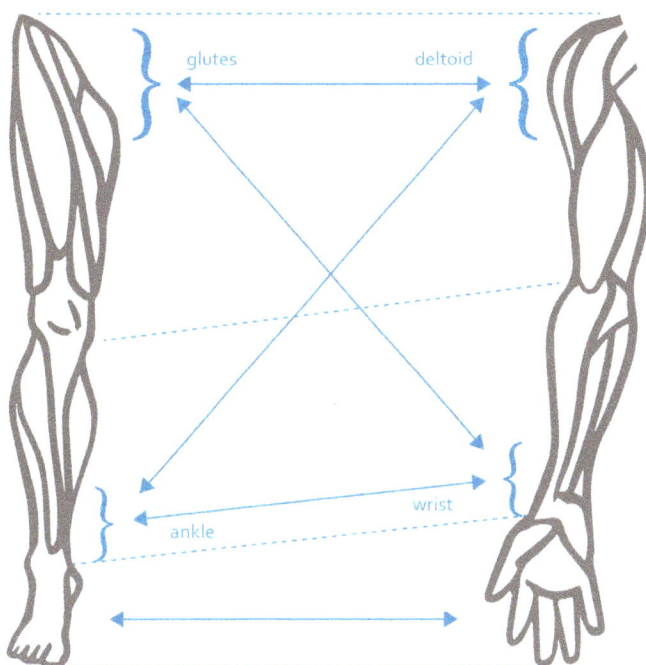

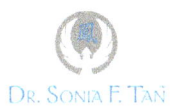

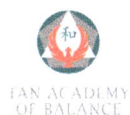

glutes   deltoid

ankle   wrist

FIGURE 9

25

ILLUSTRATIONS OF THE IMAGING CONCEPT
APPLIED IN THE BALANCE SYSTEM

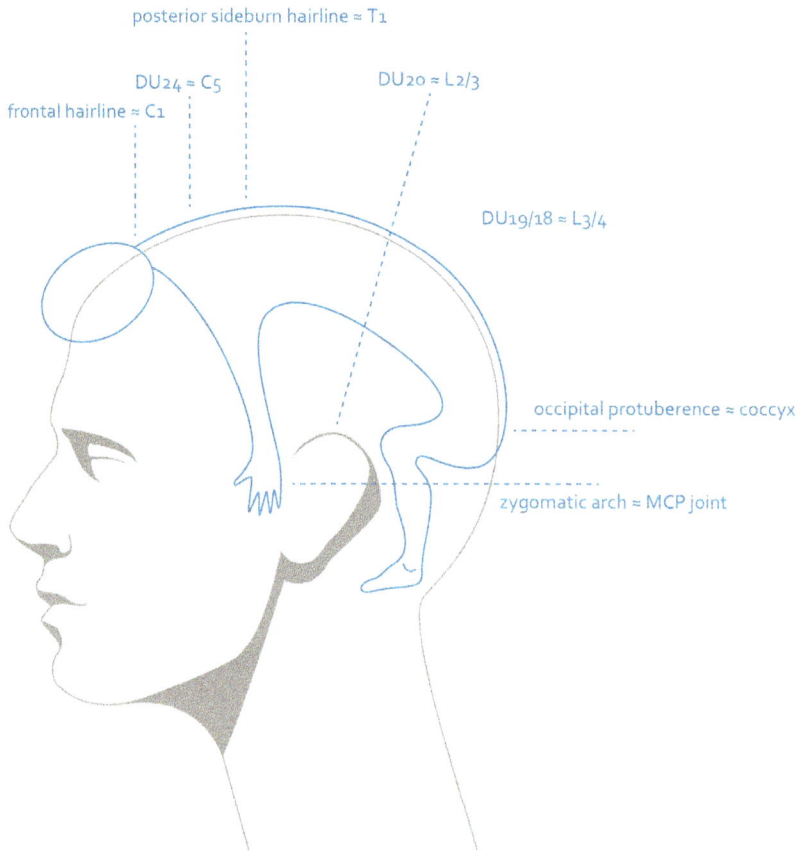

posterior sideburn hairline ≈ T1

DU24 ≈ C5

DU20 ≈ L2/3

frontal hairline ≈ C1

DU19/18 ≈ L3/4

occipital protuberence ≈ coccyx

zygomatic arch ≈ MCP joint

Dr. Sonia F. Tan

TAN ACADEMY
OF BALANCE

© Dr. Sonia F. Tan 2020

FIGURE 10

In Figure 10, you can see that the "sock monkey" or "toupee man" illustrates the use of the scalp to treat Du channel pain. Find your landmarks for the spinal segments, and feel for the change in tissue on the scalp. You can also use this area to treat Ren channel problems, such as on the chest. Just go to the corresponding spinal segment that aligns with that area.

Case Example Using System I: Míng–Name
Your patient comes in complaining of neck pain and headaches on the right side from about GB 20 down the neck to GB 21. Daily, pain is 6 on the 0–10 pain scale. What do you do?

TREATMENT: Contralateral San Jiao (Triple Heater)–Hand Shaoyang channel, using the patient's left side (in this case) and the "puppet-show" image (Figure 3) where the hand is the head, sitting on the body, which is the arm. The equivalent acupoints for GB 20 to GB 21 on this image would be approximately SJ 4 to SJ 4.75A.

NOTE: In Balance System Acupuncture, when points are followed by decimals, this is a reference for where you are on your *Āshì* 阿是 point along that channel. So 4.75 means approximately three-quarters of the way toward SJ 5. Make sense? The "A" after the number indicates you are palpated for Āshì in that area and this is an approximation of the acupoint insertion location. If you use more than one needle at that spot, then your chart notation should indicate this, by an "×" (multiplication sign) plus the number of needles. For example, SJ 4.75A × 2 means you should find the location that is approximately three-quarters of the way from SJ 4 to SJ 5, needle at this location using two needles at the palpation spots you feel the tissue change or the Qì flow blockage in the channel. Follow this nomenclature in your own chart notation, so we all speak the same language and so that you or other practitioners can understand instantly from the chart notes where you needled, and can repeat the treatment.

CHAPTER 4

The Five Steps

BEFORE YOU START NEEDLING, there are key steps to remember in order for you not only to apply Balance System Acupuncture correctly, but also to achieve better clinical outcomes. The first three steps were developed by Shīfù Tan, and is more widely known as "Acupuncture 1, 2, 3." I added two steps because I noticed there was a gap of results among colleagues and students. The last two steps that I added are important to improve patient outcomes.

The Five Steps of Balance System Acupuncture:

1. *Diagnose using Channel Theory. Which channel is sick or reflecting a blockage?* Find the sick channel. Follow the channel's flow, and assess the channels affected in area(s) of blockage where they are symptomatic.
2. *Assess which is the balancing channel?* Balance System Acupuncture contains five main systems to choose from (six in total). Determine which system you want to use. If the "sick" or blocked area is between two channels, then you must needle between the two balancing channels. Ideally, you will have an option that closely reflects this, and the two channels will be side by side. In fact, this is also the better option.
3. *Choose your acupoints by using Mirror or Image (Holography).* In the previous chapter, I provided the most widely used holographic maps in this

method (Figures 3–10). Regardless of the many more holographic maps discovered and in use, the more important thing to keep in mind is to use holographic (mirror-imaging) points in a Balance System Acupuncture way for greater clinical effectiveness and outcomes. Your best choices are using closer anatomical likeness to the affected area, and working with a wider or larger mirror-image map.

4. ***Chase the pain or discomfort level until it is at least reduced by 50 percent.*** Once you have achieved a 50 percent reduction, you know you have found the epicentre of your target treatment area. You can now avoid spending more time to achieve 100 percent reduction, as long as you follow Step 5.

5. ***Let the Qì flow for at least thirty minutes.*** Let the Qì circulate, ebb, and flow through all the channels and circuits to do its integration and processing in the body, and allow for it to complete one Qì cycle (which takes approximately twenty-nine minutes). If applied correctly, you'll likely find after thirty minutes of the Qì flow, that the majority of the remaining pain or discomfort has disappeared.

CHAPTER 5

System II: Bié-Jīng
别经/別經 (Branch–Channel)

I N THE *BIÉ-JĪNG* 别经/別經 (Branch or Variant–Channel) system, the ancients saw a relationship that came into existence when *Qì* 气/氣 was put into System I. What does it mean to put "Qì" into the system? What happens when you do? In the Chinese character for Qì 气/氣, it depicts a grain of rice being boiled and the steam that is created rises up, like a cloud or mist. The ancients realized that we can do the same with the Bā Guà. One can create steam or mist by using Fire to heat Water. Therefore, by putting the Guà symbolizing Fire on the bottom, and the Guà symbolizing Water on the top, we create steam. This Guà is unique in that the top Guà is the exact opposite to the bottom Guà, and thereby has an affinity or harmony created within itself, with the top line of the top Guà wanting to meet and be balanced with the top line of the bottom Guà, and so on (see Figure 11).

Normally, the Guà wants to go to the opposite side to create balance. But here, when it hits the "Steam Qì" Guà, it is diverted into a vertical relationship (following the natural law of steam moving vertically), and when it hits the Fire-Water Guà *Yáo* 爻 (bar line), it wants to create balance within its own Guà first (this Fire-Water Guà). So the top Yáo of the top Guà connects to the top Yáo of the bottom Guà first, and then it moves to the opposite side of the chart, following that new pathway to a different organ channel system (see Figure 11). This is System II, the Bié-Jīng–Branch or Variant–Channel) system.

Here's my trick for memorizing this tricky system: Starting with the blocked channel you've diagnosed → keep its forename → change the polarity → then switch the limbs. There you have it! As this is an even-numbered System as labelled by Shīfù Tan, the treatment side can be either ipsilateral or contralateral. For example, if the Small Intestine–Hand Taiyang channel is blocked, keep the forename (i.e., Tai), change the polarity (i.e., Yáng changes to Yīn), and switch the limb (i.e., hand becomes foot). The destination becomes the Spleen–Foot Taiyin channel. The only set of meridians you have to memorize that meet, are the middle-layered channels of Yangming and Jueyin.

SYSTEM # II

BIÉ-JĪNG 别经/別經 ➜ BRANCH-CHANNEL RELATIONSHIP

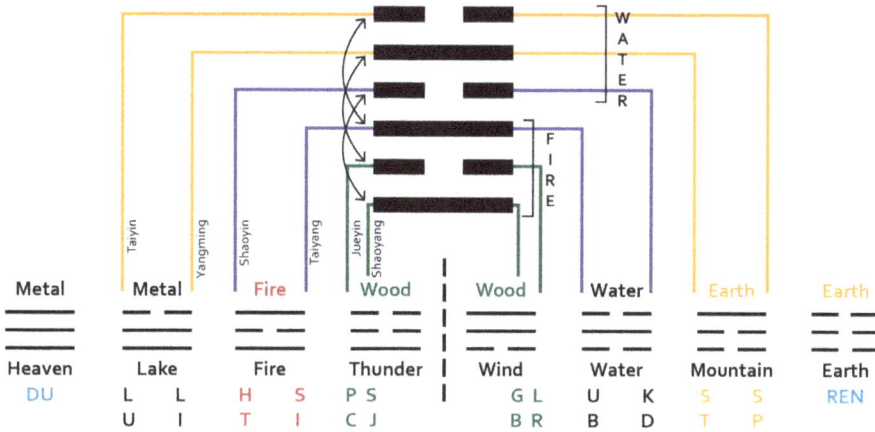

Same forename, opposite polarity.

Switch limbs.

Ipsilateral or Contralateral treatment.

© Dr. Sonia F. Tan 2020

FIGURE 11

Case Example using System II: Bié-Jīng–Branch-Channel

Your patient comes in complaining of low back pain and tension, on the left side on the Bladder–Foot Taiyang channel from about L2 to L4. Pain is 5 on the 0–10 pain scale daily. What do you do?

TREATMENT: Ipsilateral or Contralateral Lung–Hand Taiyin channel

When choosing a side, ideally you have time to palpate the patient's both arms and determine which arm has more Āshì points. If the patient is the type that doesn't feel much pain or soreness, then you must rely on your palpation skills. You should feel a tissue difference at the area that reflects the blocked area of the "sick" channel on the mirror-image map you are using—this should reflect location proportions and anatomical likeness on some maps. Examples of tissue differences are: the tissue feel knotted, ropey, nodular, tight, matted, or abnormal. Treat the limb where the tissue feels worse.

If you are using a Global Balance strategy (see the Part II), then you may not have a choice as to which side you treat. Or if your palpation skills are underdeveloped, you may not have developed a good sense yet of tissue differences and ascertaining this difference of tissue "feel" and the *Dé Qì* 得气/得氣 through the needle. If this is the case, trust that in Balance System Acupuncture, as long as you choose the correct balancing channel and correct mirror-image area, your treatment should be very effective and quick. Therefore, trust in the mirror-image locations and balancing system strategies, and needle there, feeling for good Dé Qì.

In the above case then, the corresponding acupoints would be LU 5 to LU 6A (× how many needles you've used) if you are using the Direct image, where the head is equivalent to the deltoid (Figure 3). Instead, if you used the "puppet-show" image of the body (Figure 3), where the hand represents the head, then your corresponding acupoints would be LU 4 to LU 5A (× how many needles you've used). Make sure you have *Lì Gān Jiàn Yǐng* 立竿见影/立竿見影 (set up the pole, see its shadow; instant effect), to know you have definitely found both the right channel and acupoint locations to trigger the return to balance! If you didn't achieve *Lì Gān Jiàn Yǐng*, then you have missed something, and you should go through the five steps again.

CHAPTER 6

System III: Biăo-Lĭ
表里/表裡 (Exterior-Interior)

N OW, WE MOVE INTO a time about 800 to 1,000 years later after the
first *Fú Xī Bā Guà* (Early or Pre-Heaven Sequence) arrangement. At this
time, the ancients saw a different way the Guà could be arranged to create
and illustrate harmony, and as a result, a different assignment to the organ channel
systems based on the energetics of the Guà and the organ channels. It is this era that
is most used for organ-channel Guà assignment.

The explanation for how the Guà were assigned to organ channels is best explained
in a live seminar. However, here are some easy things to keep in mind:

a) Every Guà is sitting across from its exact opposite Guà. (Look at the visual
   of the pairs of Guà in Figure 12, and you will see this relationship.) Thus,
   the Guà are in perfect harmony and illustrate this bond.

b) Each opposite pairing of Guà adds to a total of nine lines, an important number
   in *Fēng Shuǐ* 风水/風水 (geomancy) and Chinese Metaphysics.

c) Lastly, you can see these pairings are traditional partnered organ pairs taught
   in Acupuncture school. They are paired that way for a reason. And now you
   can see why—so this will be one of the easiest systems to memorize!

Because this is an odd-numbered system, treatment must be on the contralateral side, only. Try it out!

SYSTEM # III

BIĂO LǏ 表里/表裡 → EXTERIOR-INTERIOR RELATIONSHIP

(An odd number of bars is Yang, and even number of bars is Yin.)
(A Yang channel is a Yang Gua. A Yin channel is a Yin Gua.)

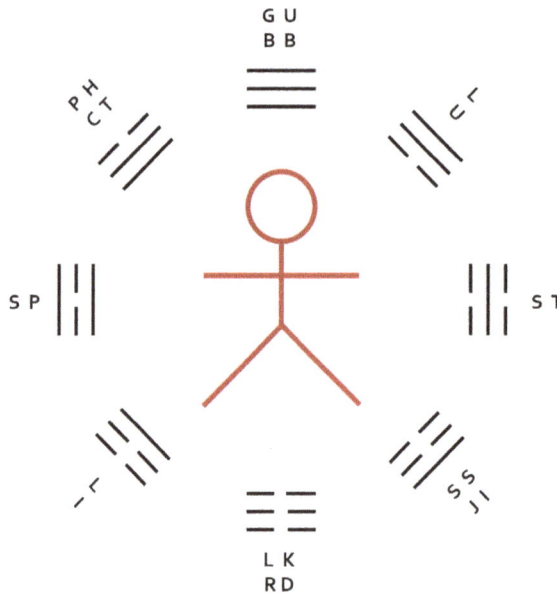

Contralateral treatment.

FIGURE 12

Case Example Using System III: Biǎo-Lǐ – Exterior-Interior

A patient comes in complaining of tibialis anterior pain and swelling on the right leg. The pain runs from approximately ST 36 to ST 41 and is quite tight and painful, a 9 on the 0–10 pain scale. The patient cannot dorsiflex their foot. What do you do?

TREATMENT: Contralateral Spleen–Foot Taiyin channel

This is potentially a humorous situation because the patient may become confused as you move toward the opposite leg. They may try to correct you and remind you which leg is injured. Just go there and explain how the Acupuncture channels often connect and balance each other using a crisscross, or contralateral, connection, just like the right side of the brain has a contralateral control mechanism—the right brain controls the left side—and show them the results in seconds!

In this case example, the corresponding acupoints would be SP 9 to SP 5A (× how many needles you've used) if you are using the direct image, where the lower leg is equivalent to the lower leg. In this situation, it is less than ideal to use a flipped image to treat the Stomach channel, since that would mean you have to use SP 10 to SP 12, an area of the body that is less convenient and safe to access.

CHAPTER 7

System IV:
Chinese Clock – Opposite

N OW WE MOVE AWAY from the *Yì Jīng* 易经/易經 (*The Book of Changes* or *I Ching*) and move into the Chinese clock. Yep, that's right, you did learn the Chinese clock in Acupuncture school for a reason!

If you lay out the Chinese clock of organ flow with the Heart channel at the noontime position (from 11 a.m. to 1 p.m.), then follow the normal organ/channel flow clockwise with each respective time, you will easily see the connection.

System IV creates balance via the opposite twelve-hour time frame—it's that simple! So, if you draw a line from the Heart to the opposite side of the circular clock, it should meet at the Gallbladder—its opposite twelve-hour time frame. The Heart's time is from 11 a.m. to 1 p.m. and the Gallbladder's time is from 11 p.m. to 1 a.m.—voilà!

In Balance System Acupuncture, remember that because this is an even-numbered system, the treatment side can be ipsilateral or contralateral.

SYSTEM # IV

CHINESE CLOCK - OPPOSITE TIME

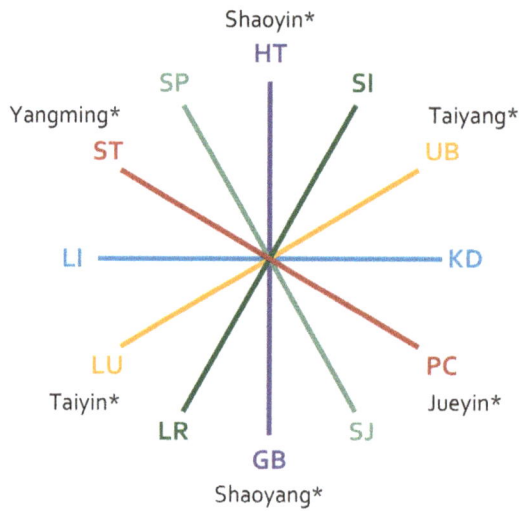

Ipsilateral or Contralateral treatment.

* End result same as System #2.

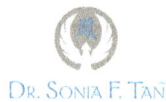

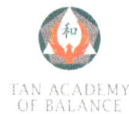

DR. SONIA F. TAN

TAN ACADEMY
OF BALANCE

© Dr. Sonia F. Tan 2020

FIGURE 13

Case Example Using System IV: Opposite Clock

A patient comes into your office complaining of scapular pain. The patient fractured their scapula in three places in a cycling accident and has pain all over the scapula. It is a 7 on the 0–10 pain scale, and the patient's range of motion is restricted. What do you do?

TREATMENT: Ipsilateral or Contralateral Liver–Foot Jueyin channel

This system is a favourite of mine and Shīfù Tan's for treating Small Intestine channel and scapular pain. The main reason for choosing the Liver channel as the balancing channel is due to the anatomical likeness. The scapula is a bony piece of anatomy, and the Liver channel is a bony channel, travelling all along the medial surface of the tibia. In addition, a practitioner can use two images on the leg to mirror the scapula. One is the puppet-show image, which places the scapula at approximately LR 4 to LR 4.75A. The other image uses the medial malleolus as a micro version of the triangular scapula, with the vertex of the scapula imaged as the proximal end of the medial malleolus. If you needle on the malleolus, choose the area that reflects the exact location of scapular pain for the patient. For example, if the patient's pain is on the superior spine of the scapula, palpate and needle the distal portion of the medial malleolus. With either image, needle across the bone subcutaneously for the most effective outcome.

CHAPTER 8

System V:
Chinese Clock – Neighbour

S YSTEM V ALSO USES the Chinese clock, but it applies a different existing balancing relationship that was discovered by the ancients.

In this system, you create balance via the neighbouring organ channel. Which neighbour? While you could look at the diagram and memorize which ones, my trick to keep it easy and work on the fly, is that the neighbour that balances the blocked organ/channel is the neighbour with the *same* polarity. So the Yīn organ channel is balanced by the neighbour that is a Yīn organ channel. That's it—another use of the clock you never thought you would ever utilize again! Remember that this is an odd-numbered system, so treatment is only on the contralateral side. Now all you have to do is visualize the Chinese clock in your head, and you can apply this system with ease!

SYSTEM # V

CHINESE CLOCK - NEIGHBOUR

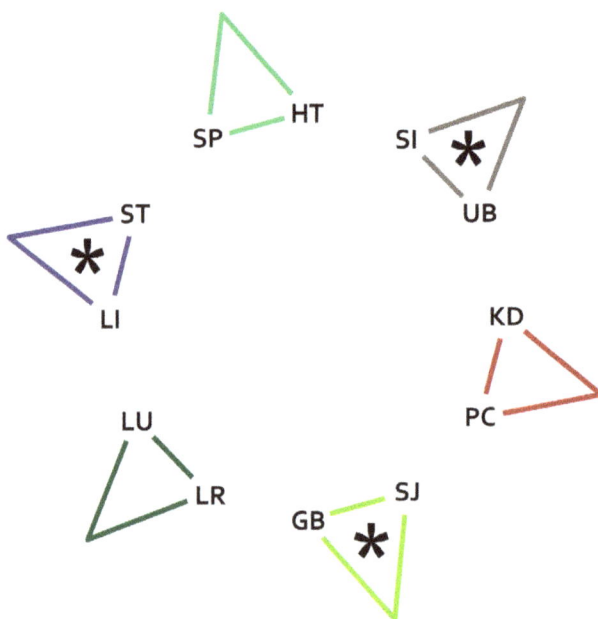

Same polarity.

Contralateral treatment.

* End result same as System #1.

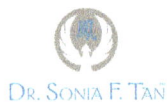

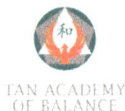

© Dr. Sonia F. Tan 2020

FIGURE 14

Case Example Using System V: Neighbour Clock

A patient comes into your office complaining of dysmenorrhea. At this point, you have only learned Single Systems Balance and not the Multiple System Balance of OBGYN 8 (which we will cover in Part II of this book). However, you can still be effective! In terms of menstrual pain, the Kidney, Stomach, and possibly Spleen channels are the main "sick" ones. What do you do?

TREATMENT: Contralateral Pericardium–Hand Jueyin channel, Contralateral Large Intestine–Hand Yangming channel, or Contralateral Heart–Hand Shaoyin channel

In this case, your best choice would be the contralateral Pericardium–Hand Jueyin channel. Not only does the Pericardium channel balance the Kidney channel in System V, but it also balances the Stomach channel in System II and IV. By choosing the Pericardium channel as the balancing channel, you are being more efficient, using one meridian to treat two channels.

In this case example, you have two choices for corresponding acupoints. One is the direct image of the Ovaries or Uterus. The Ovaries are about halfway to two-thirds down the lower abdomen, and the Uterus is about two-thirds of the way down. Therefore, on PC channel, you should be palpating and needling from PC 4 to PC 6 for dysmenorrhea. Alternatively, you can utilize a Master Tung point called *Zhōng Guān* 中关/中關 (Middle Pass/Gate) for the Uterus (and Prostate) that lies on the PC channel, at approximately PC 7.2. This acupoint is called Zhōng Guān utilizes a different mirror-image. It is similar to using Korean Hand Therapy image. Do not confuse this point as being the direct image (in which the head is the deltoid) of the Ovaries and Uterus. This Master Tung point called Zhōng Guān at the level of PC 7.2 is a great acupoint to use when you only have one needle and need to still move around.

CHAPTER 9

System VI: Hé 合 - Self

T
HE FINAL MAIN SYSTEM from the ancient classics that we use in
Balance System Acupuncture is called *Hé* 合, which means "to be identical
with" or "to adjust oneself," as used in the phrase *wěn hé* 吻合. We refer
to this system more commonly as "Self" or "Same." Here, the practitioner uses the
channel that is "sick" to treat itself. However, unlike what you learned in school, the
way we apply it is by two choices. One, you can use a mirror-image acupoint on the
meridian itself—the "sick" meridian. For example, someone sees you for mid-cheek
pain and you assess it is on the Stomach–Foot Yangming channel. Using System VI,
the point to use would be on the Stomach–Foot Yangming channel itself, and the
acupoint would be selected via the location of the cheek that has pain. Looking at
the image on Figure 5, which uses a large image of the face in a direct orientation.
The acupoint using this image would be approximately ST 40. Much of this system
is utilized in Multiple System Balance, aka Global Balance (see Part II). Or, the
second choice, my own clinical pearl—in certain cases—is the Xi-Cleft acupoints
of the self-meridian. In the above example, this would be ST 34.

Keep in mind that although this system is even-numbered, the treatment side is
only ipsilateral with this system. This is the one exception.

Case Example using System VI: Hé – Self

A patient comes into your office complaining of cheek pain, in the area of ST 3 to ST 4 and then all the way to ST 6. What do you do?

TREATMENT: Ipsilateral Stomach–Foot Yangming channel

Using the direct image of the entire face (Figure 5), the corresponding acupoints would be ST 37 to ST 40.5. If you use the flipped image of the entire face (Figure 6), the acupoints would be ST 30.5 to ST 33. If you use the mirror-image map where the foot represents the face, i.e., the puppet-show figure in Figure 4, you could also use ST 42 to ST 43. However, this choice gives you a much smaller area to work with, which makes it more difficult to accurately get at the target area.

In addition, I mentioned instead of using mirror-image points on the Self, you can use my clinical favourite, the Xi-Cleft points. In this case, it would be ST 34. In my practice, I have discovered an even better outcome: if the Xi-Cleft points are also on a mirror-image spot you are trying to heal, this may result in a double- and sometimes triple-layered effective treatment.

Research by Peter Dorsher, MD, supports the treating of the self-meridian of System VI. Looking at the commonality between myofascial lines, trigger points, and Acupuncture channels, he found that 80 percent of the myofascial lines and trigger points aligned and overlapped with Acupuncture channels (Dorsher, 2009). Furthermore, his research illustrates that when the fascia wraps around a needle, and that needle is manipulated, the tugging of the fascia at a distal level affects the entire myofascial chain (Dorsher, 2009). Muscle fibers and fascia attached to a non-coated needle more readily and comprehensively, thus enabling more of an attachment to the needle, and hence, more of a tug on the myofascial line and Acupuncture channel itself (Dorsher, 2009). I've always preferred non-coated needles, and this is further proof of their enhanced effectiveness. Effective and enhancing tools further amplify good skills.

Of course, you can still have an effect with coated needles. However, I am willing to bet you will have improved and stronger Dé Qì and clinical outcomes with non-coated needles. It is possible to educate your patient to understand that Dé Qì is good and is a desired outcome that may improve their results. They will start getting excited when you get a good one!

Other Clinical Recommendations

In addition to paying attention to the tools you are using, I want to emphasize the importance of your clinical palpation skills and your ability to feel the energetics through the needles, whether subtle or large. Remember we are holding onto a piece of metal that has been inserted into electrically charged fluid. Train your senses to feel the spark, the Dé Qì before or at the moment it happens for the patient, so that even if they don't feel it, because you are well practiced in it, you know you have the right spot of activation. This takes practice and using the best tools for you.

Lastly, about needling and needles, you will notice that when I work, I wear rings. I wear rings on my working needling hand, to protect the amount of Dé Qì I am absorbing from the patient. In the past, before I wore them, I would get pain in my metacarpal-phalangeal joints. Then taking a concept I knew growing up, I bought some jade rings for my fingers, and voilà—pain gone! You can also use quartz to help block and absorb energy. Lastly, I have found hematite helpful due to its Qì and Blood circulation properties. Happy ring hunting!

CHAPTER 10

Dr. Richard Teh-Fu Tan's Special Points

Tan Liver 8 (LR 8T)

THIS POINT IS LOCATED easiest by starting at SP 9, then moving about 1 *cùn* 寸 (unit of length or inch) anterior, and going superior onto the tibia about 2 cùn. From here, then move posterior almost to the posterior border of the tibia, and then make your way down inferiorly on the tibia about 2–3 cùn. This point is a large area, and is stimulated normally with two to three needles inserted oblique-subcutaneously. The point is the shape of a kidney bean, and the size of a credit card. See Figure 15.

INDICATIONS: Tan Liver 8 can be used as a replacement for the traditional LR 8. In Balance System Acupuncture, use it also to treat anything related to the eyes, temples, ear, conditions of the abdomen near the level of the umbilicus, and any other corresponding balancing channel it treats, as well as the mirror-image of the location.

Tan Liver 8 (LR 8T)
Dr. Richard Teh-Fu Tan's Special Liver 8 Acupoint

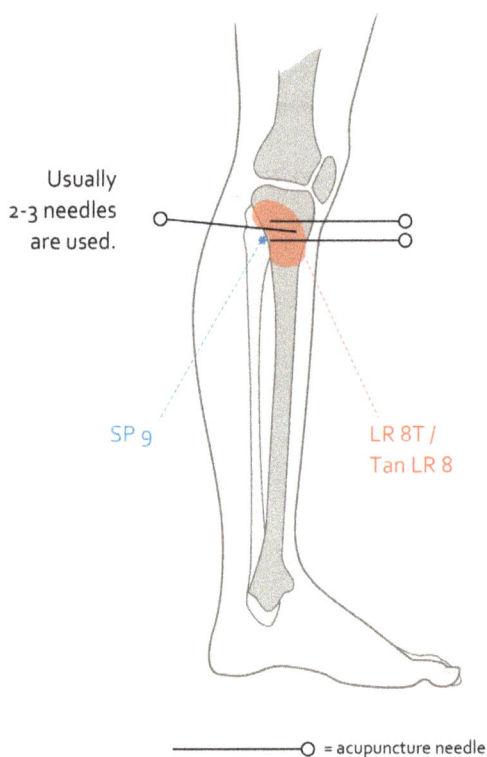

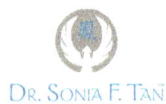

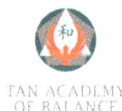

FIGURE 15

Tan Gallbladder 34 (GB 34T)

This point is located easiest by starting at the traditional GB 34, which is located at the inferior and anterior border of the fibula head. Move along the inferior border of the fibula head to the *posterior* border, and find the space *between* the bone and the tendon. If you pass the tendon and end up on the posterior side of the tendon, you have gone too far. This point tends to feel strong when needled correctly. See Figure 16.

INDICATIONS: Tan Gallbladder 34 can be used as a replacement for the traditional GB 34. In Balance System Acupuncture, use it also to treat anything related to the eyes, temples, ear, conditions of the abdomen near the level of the umbilicus, and any other corresponding balancing channel it treats, as well as the mirror-image of the location.

Tan Gallbladder 34 (GB 34T)
Dr. Richard Teh-Fu Tan's Special Gallbladder 34 Acupoint

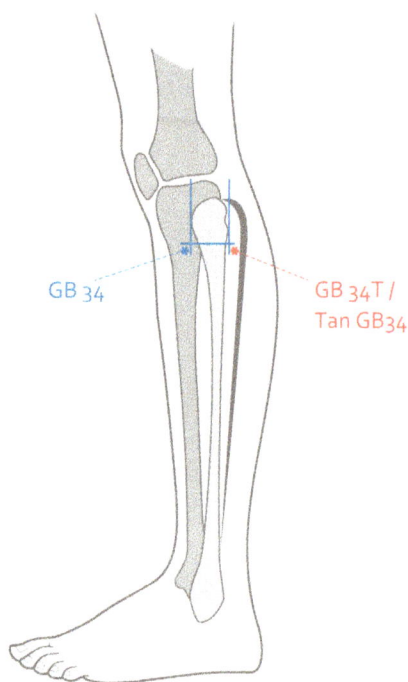

GB 34

GB 34T /
Tan GB34

FIGURE 16

PART II

Multiple Systems:
Balancing Many Channels at Once
and Internal Medicine Conditions

CHAPTER 11

Multiple Balance –
Balancing the Systems Globally

A FTER YOU HAVE JUMPED in and spent at least four weeks using only Balance System Acupuncture (Yes, jump in! Immerse to understand and observe it well!) and you have become more comfortable with its application, I imagine you are both awed and fascinated, and have more questions. That's normal! Here is where we start to get into some of your questions and move to the next level. Multiple Balance, or Global Balance, works with complex strategy and treatment plans, with broader-reaching and longer-lasting results.

The Rules of the Game: When and Why?

In multiple balance, historically coined by Shīfù Tan as Global Balance, we address three key issues – What to do if:

1. More than one area of a channel is sick.
2. More than one channel is sick, i.e. two or more.
3. A patient has internal or functional medicine problems.

This is where stronger and longer-lasting treatment steps using multiple or Global Balance are needed. Great. Where do you begin?

There are two requirements one must have to establish a Multiple or Global Balance strategy treatment where your outcomes are intended to be stronger, longer-lasting, and more broad-reaching. That last part is important to remember, because sometimes you need to your treatment to be broader, and sometimes you need to avoid this and keep specific. The two requirements come from the engineering minds of former engineers, Dr. Chao Chen and Dr. Richard Teh-Fu Tan. In fact, I come from two generations of engineers as well, so although my mind is not officially an engineer, it is informally, and I hope you appreciate it. You'll perhaps see this particularly when I teach in-person classes, and how I like to break things down, then systematically put things back together for enhanced understanding.

Requirement One: Dynamic Balance—Yīn–Yáng flow

Choose where to place acupoints according to the channel polarity and keep the polarity the same on each quadrant or limb. This creates natural law where Yīn and Yáng ebb and flow in an alternating pattern (see Figure 17).

DYNAMIC BALANCE

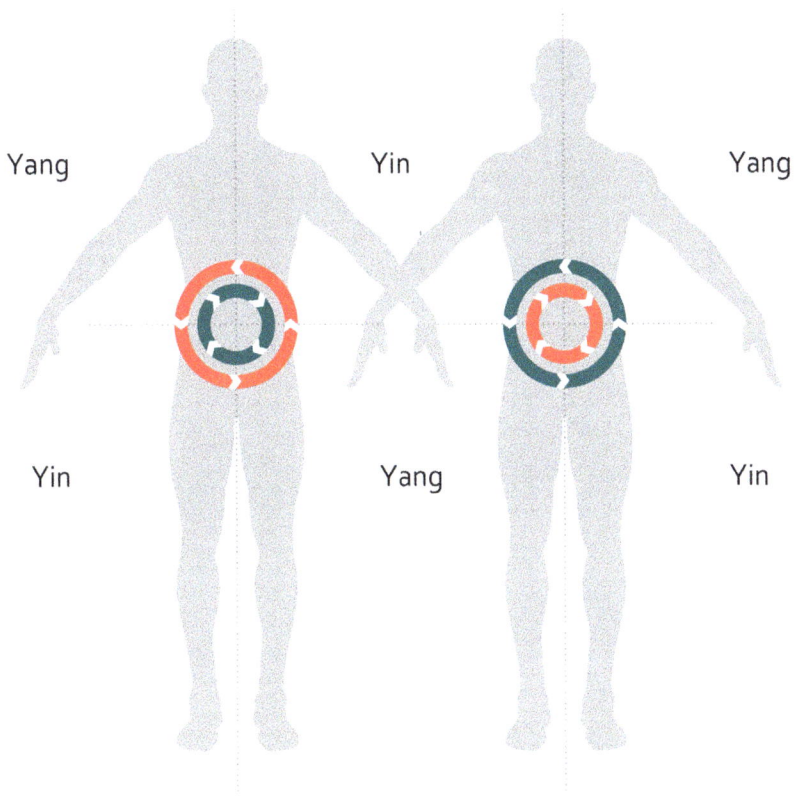

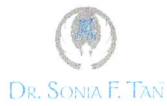

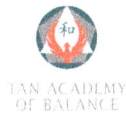

Yang

Yin

Yang

Yin

Yang

Yin

FIGURE 17

Requirement Two: Static Balance—Truss

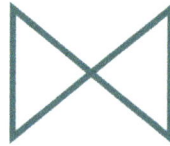

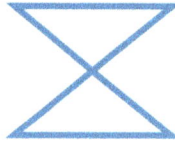

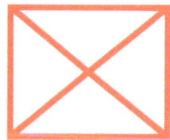

Choose which meridians to connect via the five systems of Balance System Acupuncture in order to create one of four types of engineering trusses. This is a commonly seen structure in civil engineering designed to create a strong foundation, and we use them for the same reason in Balance System Acupuncture. You do not need to have all four trusses; just one will suffice.

STATIC BALANCE - TRUSS

FIGURE 18

CHAPTER 12

The Global Balance Maps: Your Navigation Plan

I N THIS CHAPTER, I'VE included a variety of clinical "road maps" that follow Multiple or Global Balance strategies to help get you started with treatments. One thing you should keep in mind as you get started with either Shīfù Tan's or my own clinical favourites: You CAN customize within these "maps," as long as you know how to do so. I spent many classes with Shīfù Tan, and many a martini to ask and know what I could do creatively—and how he worked creatively and clinically. The customization comes with depths of knowledge of the many types of mirror-image maps and also knowing all six Single Systems well. Much of those customizations you will see come to life in class with real cases. The more customization you can do, the more focused, efficient, and improved your clinical outcomes will be. Bring it!

A few important things to mention about the "maps":

1. Any map with the name "Magic" was created by Dr. Richard Teh-Fu Tan.
2. It is not the intention of this book to explain the origin of the maps. For that information, you need to take a live seminar, which will deepen your understanding of why these maps were used and why they work.
3. The acupoints listed are the clinical favourites of Shīfù Tan. I have also shared and indicated some of my own clinical experience favourites.

4. Other "Global Balance maps" exist. In fact, in my live seminar, we cover more of these maps and also discuss how to create your own maps. In this book, I've laid out the best and most common ways to jump-start the internal medicine aspect of your practice.

5. Remember that the best treatments give the body a simple and specific message. Don't forgo using a Single Balance treatment in order to use an easy, pre-made Multiple Balance map. Multiple Balance is not always better than working with a Single Balance treatment. The more specific and streamlined the message in your treatment, the better!

A word about the term *Multiple Systems*. This is a term I developed, as a way to make more of a clear distinction and understanding of its use, function, and intended outcome. I sometimes use it interchangeably with the "Global Balance," which was coined by Shīfù Tan. My preference is to refer to it as Multiple System Balance, due to its clearer intention of utilizing two or more channels, hence systems, to achieve your clinical outcomes—whether that be for complex MSK problems or internal medicine conditions.

Million Dollar Low Back Pain Strategy ($LBP)

INDICATIONS: Low back pain on the Bladder channel primarily, requiring a stronger, longer-lasting treatment (Figure 19) where one also sees in addition to the low back pain, symptoms of leg pain or discomfort, fatigue, restlessness, and/or low energy. This collection of symptoms indicates that more than one area of the Bladder channel is blocked and that the patient may have some possible internal medicine function conditions that need to be addressed.

SIDE NOTE: Is this deficiency or just that the Qì cannot be accessed due to the blockage? Keep in mind back pain is not always due to a deficiency. In the concept of *Běn Biāo* 本标/本標 (root cause and symptoms or branch of a disease), the roots will thrive when the branches are trimmed, just like in gardening—treating the roots for the roots to thrive is not always indicated.

NOTE: Make sure you still obey the rules of Systems I–VI and its contralateral/ipsilateral requirements, and choose the proper contralateral side for the *Líng Gǔ* 灵骨/靈骨 (Spirit Bone), *Dà Bái* 大白 (Big White), *Zhōng Bái* 中白 (Centre/Middle White), Small Intestine, and Kidney channels.

Million Dollar Low Back Pain Strategy
($LBP Strategy)

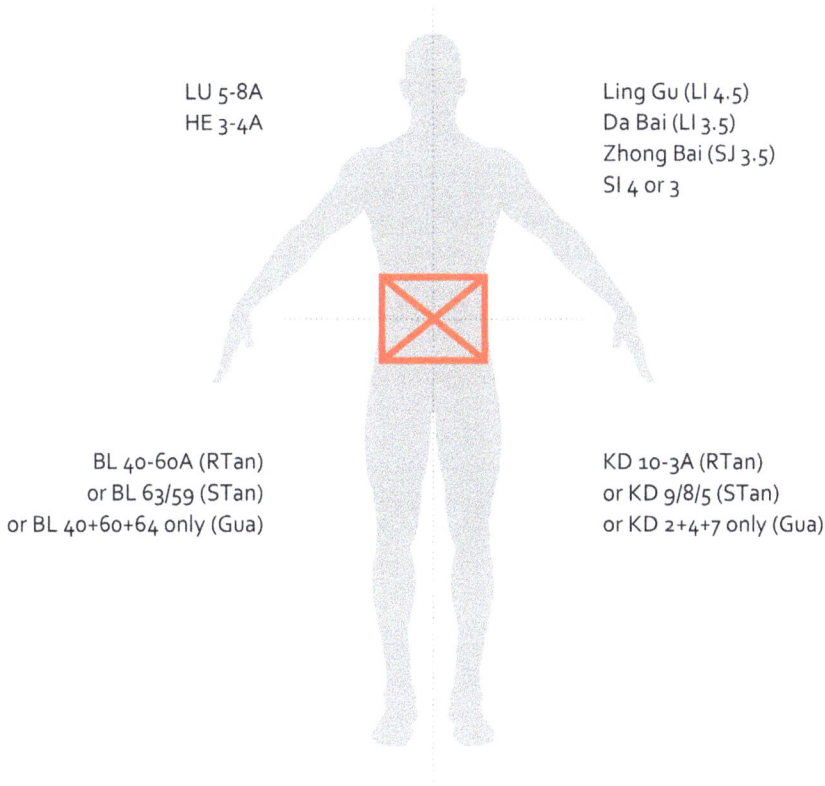

LU 5-8A
HE 3-4A

Ling Gu (LI 4.5)
Da Bai (LI 3.5)
Zhong Bai (SJ 3.5)
SI 4 or 3

BL 40-60A (RTan)
or BL 63/59 (STan)
or BL 40+60+64 only (Gua)

KD 10-3A (RTan)
or KD 9/8/5 (STan)
or KD 2+4+7 only (Gua)

Make sure you obey any contralateral rule.

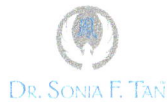

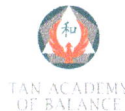

Dr. Sonia F. Tan

TAN ACADEMY
OF BALANCE

FIGURE 19

Million Dollar Low Back Pain Strategy + Gallbladder and Liver Channel ($LBP + GB + LR)

INDICATIONS: Low back pain on the Bladder channel and Gallbladder channel (see Figure 20). Remember when two or more channels are blocked, you should consider using a Multiple Balance strategy for stronger and longer-lasting outcomes.

NOTE: Make sure you still obey the rules of Systems I–VI and its contralateral/ipsilateral requirements, and choose the proper contralateral side for Líng Gǔ, Dà Bái, Zhōng Bái, Small Intestine, and Kidney channels.

Million Dollar Low Back Pain + Gallbladder and Liver Channels

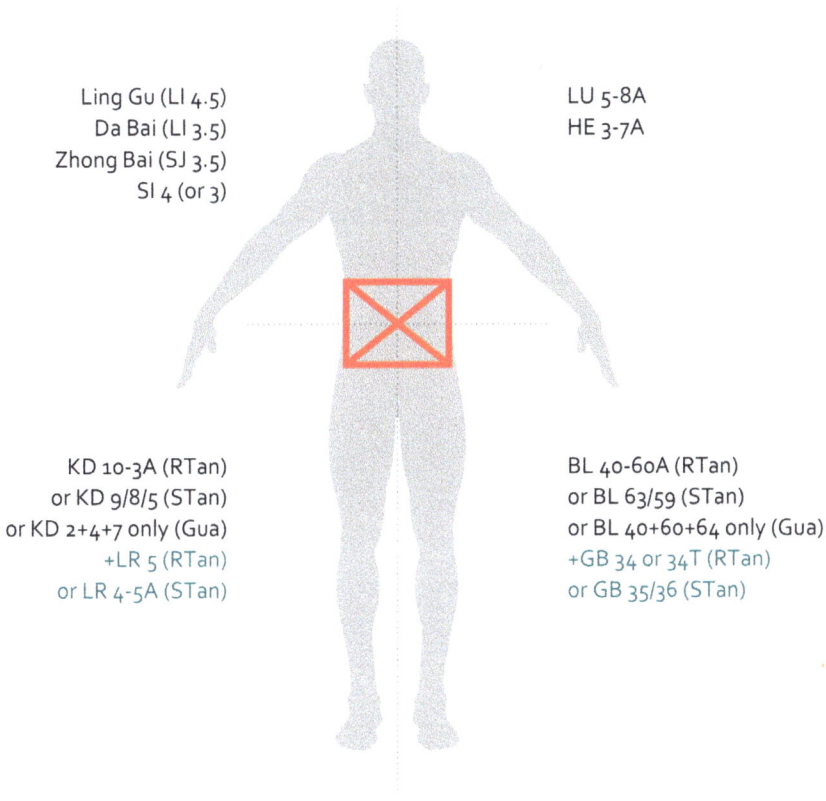

($LBP + GB + LR Strategy)

Ling Gu (LI 4.5)
Da Bai (LI 3.5)
Zhong Bai (SJ 3.5)
SI 4 (or 3)

LU 5-8A
HE 3-7A

KD 10-3A (RTan)
or KD 9/8/5 (STan)
or KD 2+4+7 only (Gua)
+LR 5 (RTan)
or LR 4-5A (STan)

BL 40-60A (RTan)
or BL 63/59 (STan)
or BL 40+60+64 only (Gua)
+GB 34 or 34T (RTan)
or GB 35/36 (STan)

*Remember to obey any contralateral rule, if warranted.

Dr. Sonia F. Tan

TAN ACADEMY
OF BALANCE

© Dr. Sonia F. Tan 2020

FIGURE 20

Magic 4 Midline Strategy

INDICATIONS: Any symptoms along the midline that includes only the Ren, Kidney, and Stomach channels (Figure 21). (The other Eight Extraordinary Vessels are not covered in this book.) The symptoms extend only as far lateral as Stomach channel. The patient uses "one hand" to show the problem. This would include chest discomfort, palpitations, gastro-esophageal reflux disease (GERD), nausea, vomiting, morning sickness, bladder conditions, and reproductive organ problems.

NOTE: Make sure you still obey the rules of the Single Systems and its contra-lateral/ipsilateral requirements. If the symptoms are unilateral, choose the proper contralateral side for those channels balancing the main sick channels of Kidney and Stomach. Also note that for women's reproductive issues, while this can be one approach, there is another one that may be appropriate. See OBGYN 8 covered later in this book.

Magic 4 Midline Strategy
(aka Magic 4 Narrow Front)
- the clinical favourite points -

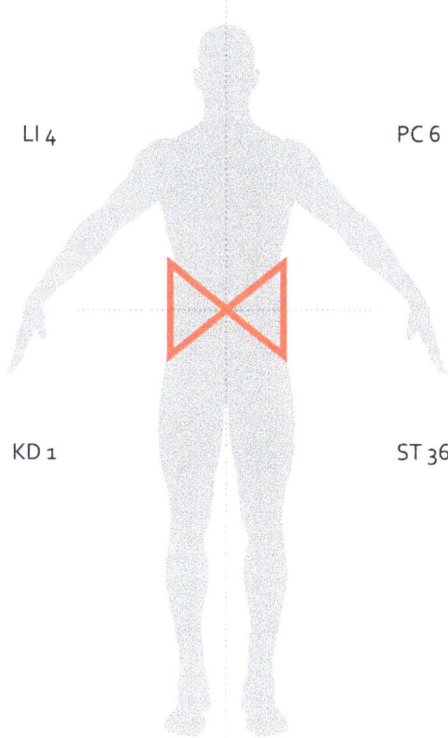

LI 4   PC 6

KD 1   ST 36

Adjust/customize as needed.
* Remember to obey any contralateral rule, if warranted.

Dr. Sonia F. Tan   TAN ACADEMY
                          OF BALANCE

© Dr. Sonia F. Tan 2020

FIGURE 21

Magic 9 (8+1) Strategy

INDICATIONS: Anything digestive where the patient's symptoms are further located lateral to Stomach channel and encompass the Spleen and Gallbladder channels (Figure 22). The patient uses "two hands" to show the problem. This would include, besides general digestive irregularities, bloating, constipation, diarrhea, irritable bowel syndrome (IBS), diabetes, and metabolic issues as examples.

NOTE: Make sure you still obey the rules of the Single Systems and its contralateral/ipsilateral requirements. Choose the proper contralateral side for those channels balancing the main sick channels, if the symptoms are unilateral.

Magic 9 (8+1) Strategy

- the clinical favourite points -

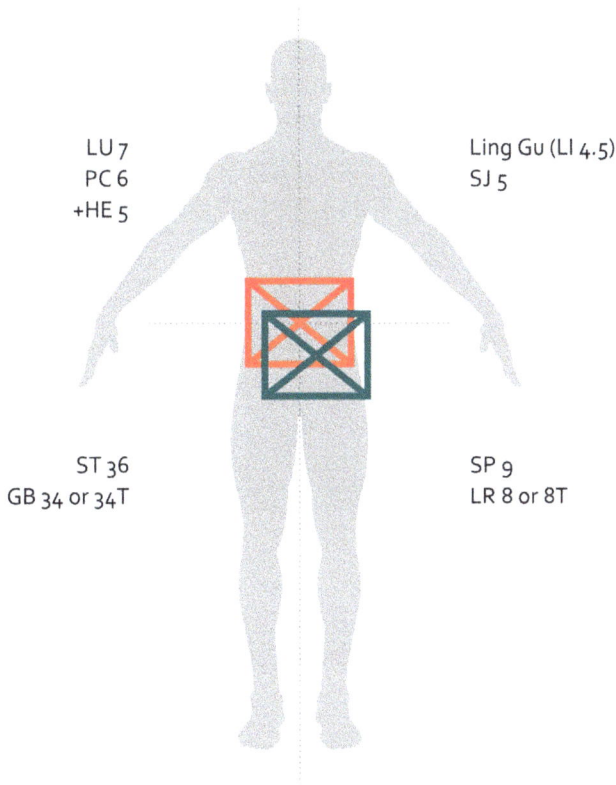

LU 7
PC 6
+HE 5

Ling Gu (LI 4.5)
SJ 5

ST 36
GB 34 or 34T

SP 9
LR 8 or 8T

Adjust/customize as needed.
* Remember to obey any contralateral rules, if warranted.

FIGURE 22

Magic 4 Heat Strategy

INDICATIONS: All types of heat, whether excess or deficient, such as infections, general deficiency-heat symptoms, fever, sweating (excess or deficient)—all heat symptoms (Figure 23).

NOTE 1: The first focus is balancing the Small Intestine channel because the SI channel is both a Fire channel and the most superficial channel in the body—the Taiyang layer. The next focus is on the Liver channel as most related to heat, because this channel is easily susceptible to heat and Fire, and this is both manifested and managed in its system flow. Thus, *when treating for heat, you should always pair the SI channel with the LR channel*, and moreover with the below Magic 4 Heat strategy as a stronger, longer lasting, internal medicine treatment.

NOTE 2: Make sure you still obey the rules of the Single Systems and its contralateral/ipsilateral requirements. Choose the proper contralateral side for those channels balancing the main sick channels, if the symptoms are unilateral.

Magic 4 Heat Strategy
- the clinical favourite points -
(non-conversion)

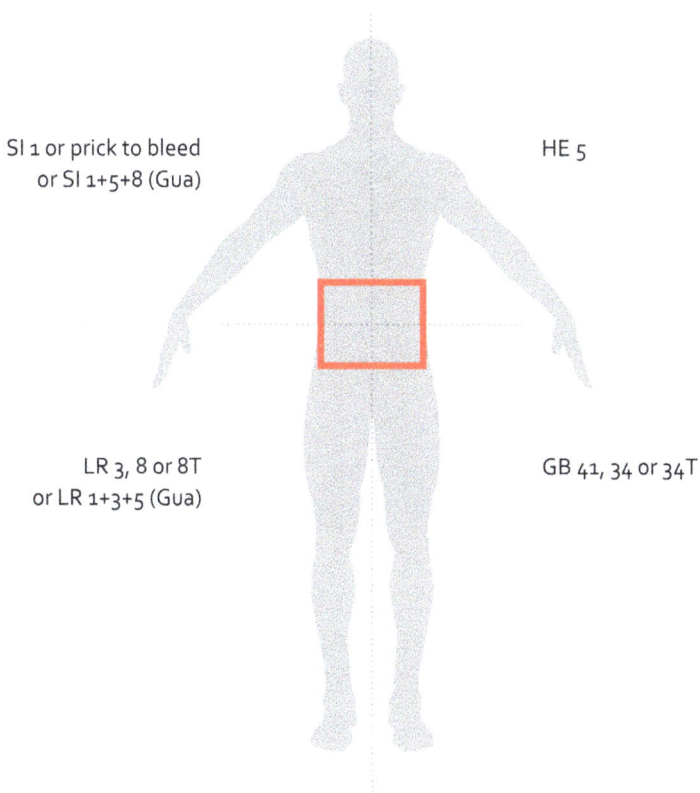

SI 1 or prick to bleed
or SI 1+5+8 (Gua)

HE 5

LR 3, 8 or 8T
or LR 1+3+5 (Gua)

GB 41, 34 or 34T

* Remember to obey any contralateral rule, if warranted.

Dr. Sonia F. Tan

TAN ACADEMY
OF BALANCE

© Dr. Sonia F. Tan 2020

FIGURE 23

Magic 4 Heat Strategy Case Example:
Real Cases from My Clinical Practice

Bruce (name changed for confidentiality) is a fifty-year-old male and one of my regular patients. He came into the clinic for an afternoon appointment, after spending the noon hour outside on one of the first warm days of spring. The temperature was 25°C (77°F), and the patient was reluctant to avoid warmth and sunshine after a long, colder than normal spring. He normally comes in for tune-ups and maintenance for his gastrointestinal health.

Today, Bruce thought he may have been out in the sun too long without any sun protection. His skin was pink and hot to the touch. He felt unwell, with symptoms of weakness and fatigue, and in the last hour, he was light-headed and dizzy, as well as nauseous. He has had sunstroke before and thought it may have been starting now. Bruce wanted to forgo the tune-up treatment and instead asked for help with these possible sunstroke symptoms. He seemed to be going downhill quickly, and his sunstroke symptoms were increasing when I put him on the table.

I needled the Magic 4 Heat clinical favourites, with the SI and LR channels treated on the left side, and the HE and GB channels treated on the right side. In this case, symptoms were widespread and bilateral. I did not need to obey a contralateral rule, so I picked the sides for the convenience of the patient's position and anatomical comfort. Within a few minutes, Bruce said he felt better, and his sensations of heat were reduced immediately. Needles were retained for a full thirty minutes. At the end of this period, Bruce said he felt back to his normal self again and the symptoms were completely resolved. He was no longer experiencing nausea or heat, his energy returned, and he was very thankful he could go home to normal evening and weekend activities.

Magic 4 Female Strategy

INDICATIONS: Women's health issues and help balancing hormones (Figure 24). This map focuses less on the physical reproductive organs, and more on women's hormones. Useful for mood regulation, irregular menstruation, night sweats, and hot flashes. (For heat symptoms, I recommend adding the two heat-regulating LR and SI organ channels, as needed.)

NOTE 1: The focus is balancing the Spleen organ channel system. It is a symbolic code in Chinese Medicine and is most strongly related to women's health as evidenced by its symptom manifestation and its functions: The Spleen produces blood, controls blood, manages bloating, and dampness (puffiness, water retention, etc.). Therefore, the Spleen is the main regulator of women's hormones.

NOTE 2: Make sure you still obey the rules of the Single Systems and its contralateral/ipsilateral requirements. Choose the proper contralateral side for those channels balancing the main sick channels, if the symptoms are unilateral.

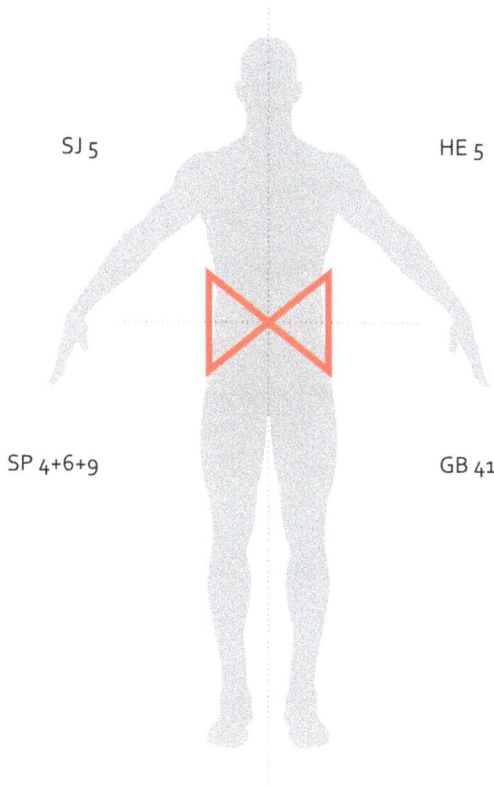

Magic 4 Female Strategy
- the clinical favourite points -
(non-conversion)

SJ 5   HE 5

SP 4+6+9   GB 41

Adjust/customize as needed.
* Remember to obey any contralateral rule, if warranted.

Dr. Sonia F. Tan   TAN ACADEMY
                          OF BALANCE

© Dr. Sonia F. Tan 2020

FIGURE 24

Magic 4 Male Strategies

This section requires more of an introduction to identify which organ channel system is most in charge of men's health. What meridian system has the most influence on male health? Liver or Kidney? Let's look at these symptoms: stagnation, courage, anger, high testosterone, urogenital flow, the inguinal region houses that the prostate, erectile function, and/or heat/hot body. This is the Liver channel and is the main one to balance male health and hormones.

If the Bladder organ is involved or the male is geriatric, then you can consider the Kidney organ/channel system as the dysfunctioning organ system instead of, or sometimes in addition to, the Liver organ/channel.

Within male hormone balancing, we have in fact, four different approaches, based on a refinement of the symptoms.

Magic 4 Male – Heat-Based Strategy

INDICATIONS: Best for men experiencing symptoms of heat, anger, irritability, or an overly hot body (Figure 25).

NOTE 1: The focus is balancing the Liver and heat. This is exactly Magic 4 Heat, which has Liver within it.

NOTE 2: Make sure you still obey the rules of the Single Systems and its contralateral/ipsilateral requirements. Choose the proper contralateral side for those channels balancing the main sick channels, if the symptoms are unilateral.

Magic 4 Male - Heat Based Strategy

-same as Magic 4 Heat -

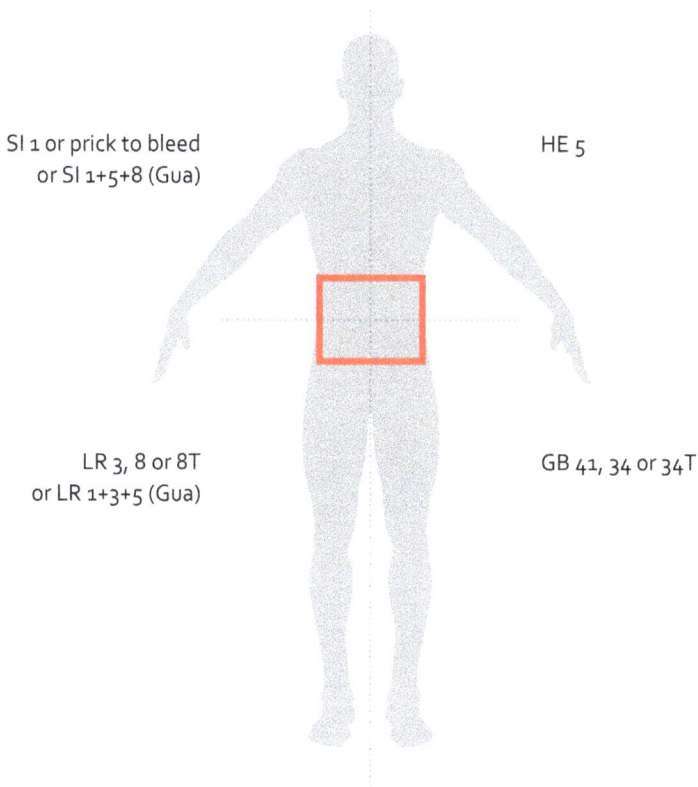

SI 1 or prick to bleed
or SI 1+5+8 (Gua)

HE 5

LR 3, 8 or 8T
or LR 1+3+5 (Gua)

GB 41, 34 or 34T

* Remember to obey any contralateral rule, if warranted.

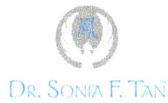

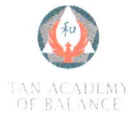

Dr. Sonia F. Tan

TAN ACADEMY
OF BALANCE

FIGURE 25

Magic 4 Male – Jueyin-Shaoyang Based Strategy

INDICATIONS: Best for when the patient has a tense / tight personality, their Pulse is Wiry, and their stress is due to having a high load of work, being overscheduled and constantly having, or needing, something to *do* (Figure 26). For example, erectile dysfunction due to stress from feeling overwhelmed. We expand more on the uses of this base in Advanced Balance System Acupuncture, Level 3: Channel-Conversion.

NOTE: The focus is balancing the Liver and Shaoyang channels. The Shaoyang channel is the navigator of linking the outside and inside world. Adjust and customize the points as needed. For example, erectile dysfunction, move the points to the wrist, hand, and fingers all the way to the tip.

NOTE 2: Make sure you still obey the rules of the Single Systems and its contralateral/ipsilateral requirements. Choose the proper contralateral side for those channels balancing the main sick channels, if the symptoms are unilateral.

Magic 4 Male
- Jueyin-Shaoyang Based Strategy -
- example points (non-conversion) for erectile dysfunction -

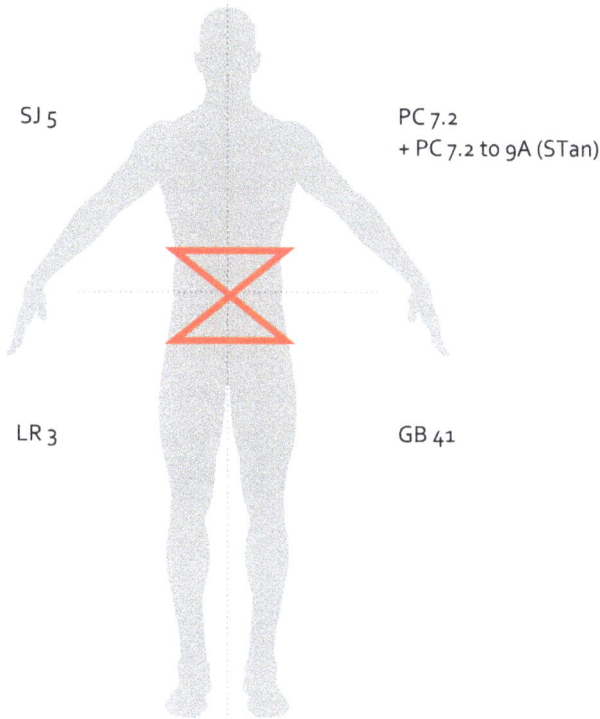

SJ 5

PC 7.2
+ PC 7.2 to 9A (STan)

LR 3

GB 41

Adjust/customize as needed. For example, add the heat
regulating pair of SI + LR channels, or Magic 4 Heat strategy.
*Remember to obey any contralateral rule, if warranted.

Dr. Sonia F. Tan

TAN ACADEMY
OF BALANCE

© Dr. Sonia F. Tan 2020

FIGURE 26

Magic 4 Male – Jueyin-Yangming Based Strategy

INDICATIONS: Best for the anxious, jittery, nervous patient, the one who constantly worries and overthinks. They tend to have a thin body and have a Thready Pulse. Their stress comes from *overthinking everything*, while also needing to do something about it. One example is erectile dysfunction due to stress from nervousness and anxiety (Figure 27). We expand more on the uses of this base in Advanced Balance System Acupuncture, Level 3: Channel-Conversion.

NOTE 1: The focus is balancing the Liver and Yangming channels. You may be confused by this idea, because your school taught you that the Spleen relates to overthinking. However, if one simply looks at Channel Theory, you can see that the Yangming channel flows on the head, and around the jaw, which functions as digesting of information, not just food. If you look further into the *Luò Mài* 络脉/絡脈 (Connecting or Network channel) trajectories, the Stomach–Foot Yangming Luò Mài flows up into the head and up to the vertex (Maciocia, 2006). Acupuncture is Channel work, and when utilized classically and appropriately, may improve both your understanding of multilayered physical, mental, and spiritual functions, and have more efficient clinical outcomes. Adjust and customize the acupoints as needed. For example, for erectile dysfunction, move the points to the wrist, hand, fingers all the way to the tip.

NOTE 2: Make sure you still obey the rules of the Single Systems and its contralateral/ipsilateral requirements. Choose the proper contralateral side for those channels balancing the main sick channels, if the symptoms are unilateral.

Magic 4 Male
- Jueyin-Yangming Based Strategy -
- example points for erectile dysfunction -

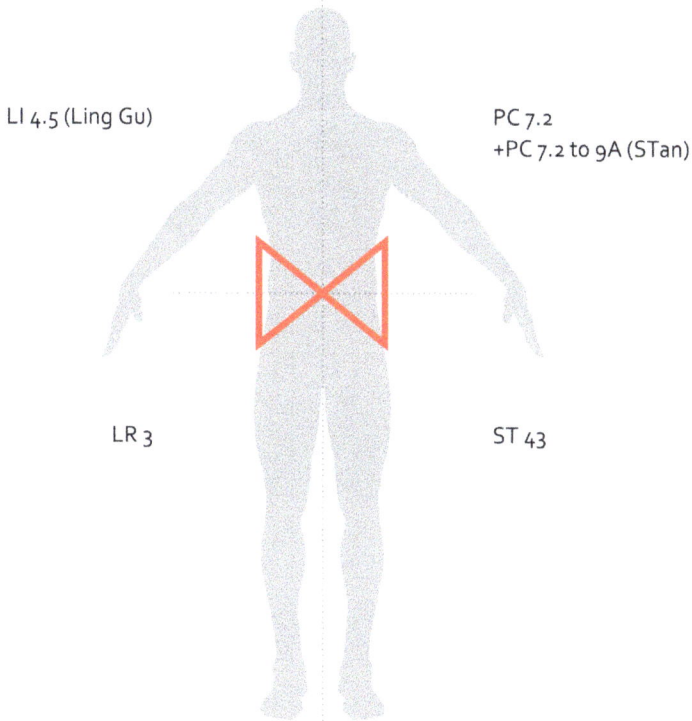

LI 4.5 (Ling Gu)

PC 7.2
+PC 7.2 to 9A (STan)

LR 3

ST 43

Adjust/customize as needed. For example, add the heat
regulating pair of SI + LR channels, or Magic 4 Heat strategy.
*Remember to obey any contralateral rule, if warranted.

DR. SONIA F. TAN

TAN ACADEMY
OF BALANCE

© Dr. Sonia F. Tan 2020

FIGURE 27

Magic 4 Male – Kidney Based Strategy

INDICATIONS: Best for when you determine the male patient's blocked channel is more the Kidney than the Liver channel. For example, the patient may have symptoms such as hypothyroidism, cold knees, and a cold back; he may be elderly, or he may have overindulged in sexual intercourse.

NOTE 1: The focus is balancing the Kidney channel. You have seen this pattern before—it is the Magic 4 Midline map. This Magic 4 Male–Kidney channel map includes the Kidney channel and the midline, which encompasses the reproductive organs. Adjust and customize the points as needed. For example, for erectile dysfunction, move the points to the wrist, hand, and fingers all the way to the tip.

NOTE 2: Make sure you still obey the rules of the Single Systems and its contralateral/ipsilateral requirements. Choose the proper contralateral side for those channels balancing the main sick channels, if the symptoms are unilateral.

Magic 4 Male
- Kidney Based Strategy -

Adjust your Magic 4 midline strategy. For example:

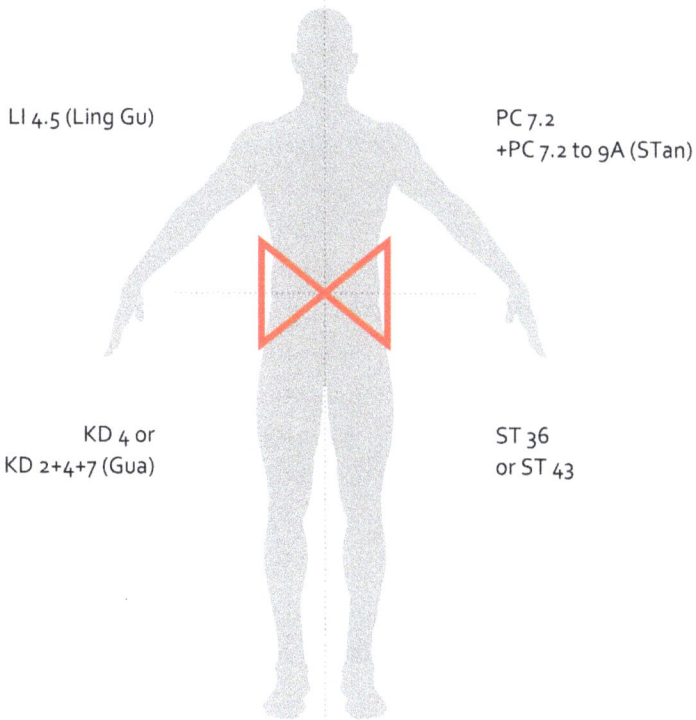

LI 4.5 (Ling Gu)

PC 7.2
+PC 7.2 to 9A (STan)

KD 4 or
KD 2+4+7 (Gua)

ST 36
or ST 43

- modified for erectile dysfunction -
* Remember to obey any contralateral rule, if warranted.

Dr. Sonia F. Tan

TAN ACADEMY
OF BALANCE

© Dr. Sonia F. Tan 2020

FIGURE 28

OBGYN 8 Strategy

When Shīfù Tan taught this "Map," like many of the previous ones, he would explain the logic of each channel chosen. I do this when I teach in-person classes. Over the years, I realized that there was an easier way to memorize this map. I asked him to verify my thinking was correct, and he nodded with assurance, "Yes, that is correct." Now when I teach, I simply introduce the map this way, as it makes more sense to me.

The Ob-Gyn 8 map or as we like to write it in Balance System Acupuncture, OBGYN 8, is simple to memorize, because it combines two maps that I have already introduced: Magic 4 Midline with Magic 4 Female. The clinical favourite points are different, however the channels are not. Remember always to focus on the channels, not the points. Shīfù Tan did say this in class and yet, somehow it often got lost or forgotten—and here is your reminder!

INDICATIONS: This map can help treat *any* obstetrics and gynecology condition (see Figure 29). Symptoms may include irregular menses, bloating, dysmenorrhea, amenorrhea, menorrhagia, endometriosis, mood swings, or irritability. This treatment can also help with cervical ripening and can be used to promote labour. I'll emphasize again, useful to treat ANY Obstetrics and Gynecology condition. Any!

NOTE 1: Make sure you still obey the rules of the Single Systems and its contralateral/ipsilateral requirements. Choose the proper contralateral side for those channels balancing the main sick channels, if the symptoms are unilateral. For example, for dysmenorrhea caused by a fibroid on one side of the body, you check exactly which channel is indicated or "sick," and obey any contralateral rule. Using the appropriate balancing channel. you can customize your treatment and do a row of Āshì points for the mirror-image of the fibroid area.

NOTE 2: Any large structural problems or physical abnormality of a certain size, as mentioned with all Balance System Acupuncture, will have limitations on how far you can achieve with your clinical outcomes, and how long it will be sustained without needing further treatment. However, you still can improve a patient's quality of life and sustain this.

OBGYN 8 Strategy

- the clinical favourite points -
(non-conversion)

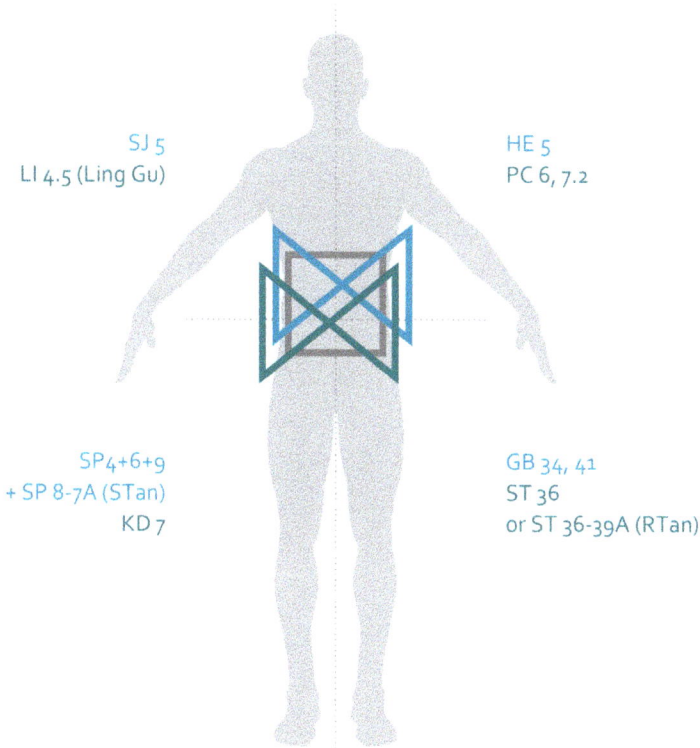

SJ 5
LI 4.5 (Ling Gu)

HE 5
PC 6, 7.2

SP 4+6+9
+ SP 8-7A (STan)
KD 7

GB 34, 41
ST 36
or ST 36-39A (RTan)

Adjust/customize as needed.
* Remember to obey any contralateral rule, if warranted.

Dr. Sonia F. Tan

TAN ACADEMY
OF BALANCE

© Dr. Sonia F. Tan 2020

FIGURE 29

SUMMARY

THE FOUNDATIONS OF BALANCE System Acupuncture are critical to master before diving into deeper tools and layers of the system. More importantly, they are essential for effective and efficient results in clinical practice. This final chapter will summarize and review some key ideas in Balance System Acupuncture. Follow these concepts to build a stronger practice and provide more effective treatments.

Key Points

The Five Steps of Balance System Acupuncture:

1. *Diagnose using Channel Theory.* Which channel is sick or reflecting a blockage?
2. *Assess which are the balancing channels?* You have five main Single balancing systems to choose from, and an additional sixth system if desired. If the area of blockage is between two channels on the balancing area, you will need to also go between those two balancing channels.
3. *Choose your acupoints by using Mirror or Image (Holography).* You have several diagrams to choose from now, and while there are more, the ones contained within this book are the most widely used. Use the mirror-imaging points in a Balance System Acupuncture way for great clinical effectiveness and outcomes.

4. ***Chase the pain or discomfort level until it is at least reduced by 50 percent*** (if treating for pain/tension/discomfort, etc.). Once you have hit the 50-percent marker, you know you have the epicentre of your target and you can avoid spending more time to find 100-percent reduction, as long as you allow for Step 5.

5. ***Let the Qì flow for at least 30 minutes.*** Let the Qì circulate, ebb, and flow through all the channels and circuits to do its integration and processing and allow for it to complete one cycle (which takes twenty-nine minutes). You'll likely find the rest of the remaining discomfort has disappeared.

Keep It Simple

Keep the message to the body as simple as possible. Avoid going to a Global Balance just because you have a pre-made "map" done for you. Think about what is in front of you: Are the symptoms truly telling you the patient needs a Multiple System balance, or can you just do a Single System balance? If you are doing a Multiple Balance, what are the least amount of meridians you need to use? Sometimes you also need to pick and choose your battle and focus on one set of symptoms first, such as the patient's chief complaint or something that includes pain. Then after a few sessions doing this, you may notice the 'other' symptoms your patient had mentioned have disappeared. When you get to a point when the main chief complaint is largely resolved, with at least three weeks of little to no symptoms, you can shift your focus. Flip to focus on other things, while still having some points or a Multiple Balance strategy, for continued correction of the original chief complaint.

Educate your patient on this transition from the beginning, about how the treatment will progress. Tell the patient that you will start by addressing the chief complaint, will reassess after a good course of treatments (most cases at least a few weeks), and will continue to target any remaining complaints until most symptoms have abated for at least two to three weeks. At this point, they will likely no longer require corrective treatments and have "mini-graduated" from the majority of any symptomology (none for at least two weeks in most cases). The last stage is their "full graduation" where they are only on a "maintenance" or "tune-up" schedule, usually at least every season (most are about every four to six weeks).

When to Think Globally

When two or more meridians are blocked, or one channel is affected on many areas throughout the channel, then you may need to consider a Multiple System balance strategy, therefore a stronger or longer-lasting treatment. Single balance will still work, but a Multiple balance will work even better—creating a more efficient and longer-lasting treatment. Lastly, whenever there is a functional or internal medicine issue, you must use a Multiple Balance approach.

Lì Gān Jiàn Yǐng 立竿见影 – Stand the Pole, See Its Shadow.

If you do not see "instant" results (e.g., in pain level, discomfort, tension, or range of motion), you may have not applied the method correctly. Check to see what you may have done incorrectly. Ask yourself the following questions: *What have I missed? Did I miss diagnosing a channel that is sick? Did I use the correct balancing meridian, or not? Did I translate and apply the correct mirror or image location?* If you check your steps and feel you did everything correctly, you should suspect that the patient may have a physical abnormality or deformity that cannot be reversed. This is for you to be more informed as well as to educate the patient. If the patient does have this sort of abnormality, make sure to communicate an accurate perspective of how far you can get with the treatments. Avoid giving up! Keep going. You can often still reduce pain levels significantly, to a 1 or 2 on the 0–10 pain (or discomfort) scale, which will improve the patient's quality of life.

Remember that Balance System Acupuncture can treat more than pain. Your treatments can restore function, promote cellular healing, and restore the proper state of balance in the body. You are promoting where the body should normally be, and function in harmony.

Mirror-Images

Get to know the mirror-images well (see Figures 3 to 10). You can utilize and layer many mirror-images on one area you are needling and be more efficient with your needling. For example, treating both low abdomen and the forehead? Use the forearm or the leg, where you employ both the flipped head image and the direct body image. If the blocked area is between two channels, when treating the balancing area, needle between the two balancing channels on areas as close to an anatomical likeness as possible. Always try to needle the reflected blocked area you want to transform.

Many more mirror-images exist. If you choose to research more mirror-images, my recommendation is you use them in a Balance System Acupuncture format for more effectiveness. Shīfù Tan researched many mirror-images and created multilayered treatments with powerful outcomes. If you choose not to research more mirror-images, that's fine, too—you don't have to find more images. I've used much of these main mirror-images (as provided in this book) in my practice and not many additional ones, for more than fifteen years. As long as you are good at channel diagnosis, can identify the appropriate balancing channel or "Map", translate what mirror-image to use, and strengthen your palpation and needling Dé Qì skills, you will have amazing results! I do, as well as many other practitioners of this style of acupuncture.

The Road Maps

Dr. Richard Teh-Fu Tan thoroughly put together and tested out the pre-designed "Magic Maps." Use them as your navigation plan and to help you start an effective practice. Remember what I have said: You can be even more effective by customizing within these "Magic Maps." As long as you know the rules of the game, you can play well within them.

What's Next?

Once you learn the techniques in this book, and use them well to achieve good results with your clients, you may want to deepen your knowledge and your practice with Advanced Balance Acupuncture coursework. For instance, if you want to use Balance System Acupuncture to treat mental health issues and internal medicine (such as immunity or stress-related Irritable Bowel Syndrome (IBS), you can take the Level 3: Channel-Conversion. Everything and everywhere is affected in the patient? Take the Level 4: The Twelve Meridian System seminar. Level 5 covers Five Phase Balancing (i.e., Five Element) problems, and Level 6: Balance in the Seasons is for those conditions that occur annually or seasonally. After that, you're at another level and further advanced classes discuss combining strategies without breaking rules and address difficult, complex cases.

While your journey could end with Balance System Acupuncture alone, you could continue to dive into the other essences of Chinese metaphysics such as *Fēng Shuǐ* 风水/風水 (geomancy) and Chinese Astrology, which were all classically practiced by the doctors of ancient China. For example, you could learn how to integrate the use of a Chinese Astrology chart into an Acupuncture session or lifestyle and diet choices, creating a truly specific and customized health plan. You also could explore learning Fēng Shuǐ and be able to advise to some extent on the patient's home environment. Another valuable area of Channel Theory you may want to incorporate into your practice picture is learning the Eight Extraordinary Vessels and Luo Channels in depth, and how to integrate them in a Channel Theory way. Understanding these vessels can help you dive deeper into the psycho-emotional and psycho-spiritual aspects of the body. This may help you treat conditions such as trauma and deep unresolved grief, or help a patient cope with life transitions, etc. A whole new world will open up in your practice and for your patients.

Regardless of how you choose to journey, I encourage you to simply do that—journey, move forward. Ask questions. Join me in person. I'm here for you when you need me. Join another teacher's classes if you wish another perspective. Throughout your journey, remember to grow, layer, and transform. This is how the medicine keeps going, survives, and evolves. Enjoy the ride.

—*Dr. Sonia F. Tan*, BA, BA(H), DAOM, R.Ac., R.TCM.P.

GLOSSARY

The terms below are those mentioned in the book, with the exception of the Acupuncture channel names. Terms are listed in alphabetical pinyin order.

Pinyin	Simplified Chinese	Traditional Chinese	English
Āshì	阿是	阿是	Literal: "Ah yes" Point of most tenderness
Bā Gāng Biàn Zhèng	八纲辩证	八綱辯證	Eight Principles
Bā Guà	八卦	八卦	Eight Symbols Eight Trigrams Eight Hexagrams
Bèi Jí Qiān Jīn Yào Fāng	备急千金要方	备急千金要方	*Essential Prescriptions Worth a Thousand in Gold for Every Emergency*
Běn Biāo	本标	本標	Root cause and symptoms or branch of a disease
Biǎo-Lǐ	表里	表裡	Exterior-Interior
Bié-Jīng	别经	別經	Branch–Channel

Pinyin	Simplified Chinese	Traditional Chinese	English
Cān Tóng Qì	参同契	参同契	*The Seal of Unity of the Three* aka *Akinness of the Three*
Cùn	寸	寸	Unit of measurement or inch
Dà Bái	大白	大白	Big White
Dé Qì	得气	得氣	Arrival of Qi (obtaining needling sensation)
Dì	地	地	Earth
Fēng Shuǐ	风水	風水	Literal: "Wind-Water" Geomancy
Fú Xī	伏羲	伏羲	The first mythical Chinese emperor
Fú Xī Bā Guà	伏羲八卦	伏羲八卦	Early Sequence Bā Guà Pre-Heaven Sequence Bā Guà
Hé	合	合	Self (To be identical with; To adjust oneself)
Huáng Dì Nèi Jīng	黄帝内经	黄帝內經	*The Yellow Emperor's Internal Medicine Classic*
Jīng-Luò	经络	經絡	Channel Meridian Pathway Route channel Connecting or Network
Lì Gān Jiàn Yǐng	立竿见影	立竿見影	Set Up a Pole and See the Shadow; instant effect
Líng Gǔ	灵骨	靈骨	Spirit Bone

Pinyin	Simplified Chinese	Traditional Chinese	English
Luò Mài	络脉	絡脈	Connecting channel Network channel
Míng	名	名	Name
Qì	气	氣	Qi
Quán Xī	全息	全息	Holographic Microsystem
Rén	人	人	Humankind
Rú shěn zāo féng zhāng dì èr shí wǔ	如审遭逢章第二十五	如審遭逢章第二十五	*Chapter 25: Examination of Suffering*
Sān Cái	三才	三才	Three Essences
Shǎo Yáng	少阳	少陽	Diminished Yang
Shǎo Yīn	少阴	少陰	Diminished Yin
Shīfù	师傅	師傅	Master (honorific)
Tài Jí	太极	太極	Supreme Ultimate
Tài Yáng	太阳	太陽	Greater Yang
Tài Yīn	太阴	太陰	Greater Yin
Tǐ Yìng Quán Xī	体应全息	體應全息	Tissue Correspondence Holographic Model
Tiān	天	天	Heaven

Pinyin	Simplified Chinese	Traditional Chinese	English
Wěn hé	吻合	吻合	Coincide Match Be correspondent
Wén Wáng Bā Guà,	文王八卦	文王八卦	King Wen Bā Guà Later Sequence/ Arrangement Bā Guà Post-Heaven Sequence/ Arrangement Bā Guà
Wú Jí	无际	無際	Primordial universe
Wǔ Xíng	五行	五行	Five Phases Five Elements
Xiè xiè	谢谢	謝謝	Thank you
Yáng	阳	陽	Yang
Yáo	爻	爻	Bar lines
Yì Jīng	易经	易經	*The Book of Changes* *The I Ching*
Yīn	阴	陰	Yin
Yuán Qì	原气	原氣	Original Qi Ancestral Qi
Zàng Fǔ	脏腑	臟腑	Organ(s)
Zhōng Bái	中白	中白	Centre/Middle White
Zhōng Guān	中关	中關	Middle Pass Middle Gate

REFERENCES

Alfaro, A. (2014, August 24–27). How to balance for otitis uveitis nasal congestions sinusitis and Internal Disorders. XVI International Conference on Traditional Chinese Veterinary Medicine, Chiayi, Taiwan.

Chen, C., Y. Chen, & D. Twicken. (2003). *I Ching Acupuncture.* California: I Ching Acupuncture Center.

Deadman, P., & M. Al-Khafaji. (2000). *A Manual of Acupuncture.* East Sussex: Journal of Chinese Medicine Publications.

Dharmananda, S. (2001). *Sun Simiao: Author of the earliest Chinese encyclopedia for clinical practice.* http://www.itmonline.org/arts/sunsimiao.htm

Dorsher, P. T. (2006). Trigger Points and Acupuncture Points: Anatomical and Clinical Correlations. *Medical Acupuncture 17*(3): 20–23

Dorsher, P. T. (2008). Optimal localization of acupuncture points: implications for acupuncture practice, education, and research. *Medical Acupuncture 20*(3): 147–150.

Dorsher, P. T. (2009). Myofascial meridians as anatomical evidence of acupuncture channels. *Medical Acupuncture 21*(2): 91–97.

Longhurst, J. C. 2010. Defining meridians: A modern basis of understanding. *Journal of Acupuncture and Meridian Studies 3*(2): 67–74.

Pregadio, F. (2011). The Seal of the Unity of the Three. In S. 66-67, *The Seal of the Unity of the Three* (p. 107). Mountain View, CA: Golden Elixer Press.

Tan, R.T-F. (2003). *Dr. Tan's Strategy of Twelve Magical Points.* San Diego: Richard Tan.

Tan, R.T-F. (2007). *Acupuncture 1,2,3.* San Diego: Richard Tan.

Tan, R. T-F. & S. Rush. (1994). *Twenty-Four More in Acupuncture: Advanced Principles and Techniques.* San Diego: Richard Tan.

Tan, R. T-F. & S. Rush. (1996). *Twelve and Twelve in Acupuncture: Advanced Princples and Techniques.* (2nd ed.) San Diego: Richard Tan.

Tan, S. F. (2004–2015). Balance Method: Core Foundations, Advanced Track and Three Essentials courses. North America.

Tan, S. F. (2004–2020). Balance Method courses and Balance System Acupuncture teachings of Sonia F. Tan. North America.

Tan, S. F. (2010–2011). *Classical Feng Shui practitioner certification training with Marlyna Los.* Vancouver: Marlyna Los.

Tan, S. F. (2016). A retrospective case series analysis on a novel acupuncture and Traditional Chinese Medicine diagnostic and treatment approach, and its efficacy results in treating allergic rhinitis [Doctoral capstone project, Yo San University, Los Angeles]. https://yosan.edu/wp-content/uploads/2018/11/Novel-Traditional-Chinese-Medicines-results-in-treating-Allergic-Rhinitis-by-Sonia-F-Tan.pdf

Travell, J. G., & D. G. Simons. (1982). *Myofascial Pain and Dysfunction: The Trigger Point Manual.* (Vol. 1). Baltimore, MD: Williams & Wilkins.

Travell, J. G., & D. G. Simons. (1983). *Myofascial Pain and Dysfunction: The Trigger Point Manual.* (Vol. 2). Baltimore, MD: Williams & Wilkins.

Twicken, D. (2012). *I-Ching Acupuncture: The Balance Method.* London: Singing Dragon.

Young, W. C. (2008). *Lectures on Tung's acupuncture therapeutic system.* San Francisco, CA:: American Chinese Medical Culture Center.

Young, W-C., C. W. Chang, & W.R. Morris. (2003). *The theory and application of ti ying quan xi (tissue correspondence holographic model).* Korea: Korea.

Young, W-C. (2006). Dr. Young & Tung's Acupuncture. http://www.drweichiehyoung.com/dr-young-tungs-acupuncture

ABOUT THE AUTHOR

Dr. Sonia F. Tan, BA, BA(H), DTCM Dip, DAOM, R.Ac., R.TCM.P., has been helping guide people on their pathway to health in the TCM world since 2006. She is a Doctor of Acupuncture and Oriental Medicine (DAOM degree), a Registered Acupuncturist (R.Ac.), and a Registered Traditional Chinese Medicine (TCM) Practitioner (R.TCM.P.). She obtained her clinical research doctorate degree from Yo San University of Traditional Chinese Medicine in Los Angeles, California and was the recipient of the DAOM Distinction Award (for excellence in clinical research and clinical didactic work). Her research was on "A novel approach to treating Allergic Rhinitis and its efficacy results." She is also a graduate of the five-year Doctor of Traditional Chinese Medicine program from the International College of Traditional Chinese Medicine of Vancouver. Dr. Sonia F. Tan is one of few certified Gold-level practitioners of the late Dr. Richard Tan, and she was personally given permission by him to call him *Shīfù* 师傅/師傅 (honorific Master). She studied the Balance Method with Dr. Richard Teh-Fu Tan from 2004 until his passing in 2015. His most advanced level courses after all Balance Method levels, were first completed by a group of sixteen senior students. Dr. Sonia F. Tan was one of those sixteen. With the blessings of fellow direct senior students to pass on the Balance Method legacy, she developed and created the very first Balance Method/System Acupuncture Certificate program at an accredited public post-secondary institution—Langara College in Vancouver—launched in 2018.

In 2010, Dr. Sonia F. Tan was honoured to be named and be a part of the Vancouver 2010 Olympic and Paralympic Medical Teams. She has been teaching and delivering keynote speeches since 2013 and has been a guest on numerous media shows. She has also completed many adjunct and advanced therapy courses, such as Sound Healing, TCM Clinical Aromatherapy and Essential Oils, and Drs. Jeffrey Yuen and

Yvonne Farrell's Eight Extraordinary Vessels approach, that she continually uses in her practice.

In addition, following in her grandfather's footsteps and the classical umbrella of Chinese Medicine, Dr. Sonia F. Tan has completed apprenticeships in Chinese Metaphysics in the areas of Chinese Astrology, Face Reading, and Classical *Fēng Shuǐ* 风水/風水 (geomancy). She completed these certifications under various teachers in 2011. She is a direct and first graduating class disciple of the late Grandmaster Dr. Richard Teh-Fu Tan and certified in Bā Zì 八字 (Eight Characters or Symbols) Chinese Astrology. She has also trained with, and is a certified Fēng Shuǐ and Chinese Astrology practitioner since 2011 under Master Marlyna Los. As a student of a variety of martial arts since 1995, Dr. Sonia F. Tan is grateful to her Shīfù the late Dale Johns, for her foundation, and to Shīfù Matthew Dyck for continuing to guide her along this path.

Dr. Sonia F. Tan is grateful to her patients, practice, and her award-winning clinic in Vancouver, BC, Canada. Following in the footsteps of both her grandfathers, Sonia is immersed in all aspects of Chinese Metaphysics, and thoroughly enjoys educating and inspiring others!

ABOUT THE FOREWORD AUTHOR

John Mini, MScM, L.Ac., is a licensed acupuncturist and herbalist who has lived and worked in the San Francisco Bay area, California, since 1988. He began studying Chinese Medicine and Taoist philosophy and the beliefs and sciences of indigenous cultures at a very early age and has always maintained his enthusiasm in these areas. Along with his acupuncture practice, he has studied and used his knowledge of indigenous and modern sciences to discover how best to help his patients. He was one of Dr. Richard Teh-Fu Tan's senior students and has utilized the Balance Method since his first meeting with Shīfù Tan in the mid-1990s. John is one of Shīfù Tan's "First Sixteen" and Certified Gold Level Practitioners. The results of his research and experience had led him to writing, nonprofit work, leading seminars and workshops to help more people than he's able to treat in his private medical practice. John Mini is also the author of the book *Marijuana Syndromes: How to Balance the Effects of Cannabis with Traditional Chinese Medicine.*

www.ingramcontent.com/pod-product-compliance
Lightning Source LLC
Chambersburg PA
CBHW041911220326
R18017400001B/R180174PG41597CBX00006B/5